Geoff Phillips is a retired Liverpool Teaching Hospital Consultant Geriatrician who for some 25 years was in increasing demand as a Medico-legal Expert. Throughout his career in medicine (and before) he observed life, and collected an archive of stories reflecting pathos, humour and the oddities of life together with interesting facts. He used some of them to enhance student and postgraduate teaching on his ward rounds and also when giving "after dinner speeches". The book is drawn from that archive and adapted for the general audience.

Acknowledgments

I would like to acknowledge the support and encouragement which I have received from friends, family and colleagues from many disciplines who have encouraged the writing of this book. Many have provided material which expanded the archive from which this book was written. Unfortunately, much of the material comes from sources unknown. I can thank the Daily and Sunday Telegraph for having supplied oddities and their letter page is always inspiring. My copy of The Chronicle of the 20th Century has allowed me to check the timings of historic events and the numerous reliable sources available on the internet, particularly Wikipedia have allowed me to "flesh out" some issues. Special thanks are owed to my secretary/PA, Mrs Patricia Hunt, for her suggestions, speed and accuracy in typing up this book in addition to my medico-legal reports. Last but not least the wonderful publishing team at Austin Macauley deserve the credit for making it actually happen, I thank you all.

Dedication

This book is primarily dedicated to the family. Firstly, to my dear wife Linda, whose unfailing support through the thick and thin of life, since we met in 1973, has been above and beyond the call of wifely duty – the epilogue illustrates examples of her forbearance. Our three daughters deserve gratitude for their numerous tolerances not least of all for my mention of indiscretions also in the epilogue.

Dr. Geoff Phillips

GNOMIC WISDOM

AUSTIN MACAULEY
PUBLISHERS LTD.

A CIP catalogue record for this title is available from the British Library.

ISBN 9781786129154 (Paperback)
ISBN 9781786129161 (Hardback)
ISBN 9781786129178 (E-Book)
www.austinmacauley.com

First Published (2017)
Austin Macauley Publishers Ltd.
25 Canada Square
Canary Wharf
London
E14 5LQ

Prologue

Contrary to the title, this book has nothing whatsoever to do with gnomes. The cover features a picture of six gnomes accompanied by a stethoscope, a Barrister's wig and an RAMC cap badge, which have great significance, indicating some forty-four years of involvement with medicine, a ten year career with the Territorial Army and over twenty-five years of experience in preparing medico-legal reports.

The gnomes, however, have some minor significance. Those in the picture were presented to me, upon my retirement from the NHS in 2011, as a reminder of a tale I once told to junior doctors on a ward round. The then Registrar of the 'Firm', had done well for himself, had become a Consultant Geriatrician and at the time of my retirement, was Clinical Director.

The tale in question relates to my involvement on a domiciliary visit with an elderly lady who had early, but unrecognised and undiagnosed, Lewy Body dementia. In simple terms, Lewy Body dementia is one of the sub-groups of dementia in which signs and symptoms of Parkinson's disease feature. They are also particularly prone to hallucination, especially if given anti-Parkinsonian drugs such as Sinemet or Madopar. This is what in fact had happened. Her General Practitioner had seen the pill-roll tremor, the slow shuffling gait and the slowness of movement and diagnosed Parkinson's disease. He then prescribed, as was normal for the time, a trial of Sinemet. Almost immediately there were profound hallucinations, which resulted in my being asked to see her at home. When I visited, she was sitting in an armchair in front of the fire, pointing at the alcoves on either side of the hearth. There were two distinct families of gnomes, one family were living in the left alcove and another family living in the right. They were in fact neighbours, and got on reasonably well but in the meantime, in front of her, they were acting out all their daily lives, washing, cleaning, cooking, eating, making love and often bickering. They were there all her waking hours and causing her a great deal of distress. When anyone visited, she pointed them out and asked the visitor to get rid of them.

I decided that it would be worth admitting her for a period of observation, cessation of the Sinemet and perhaps a trial of one of the newer antipsychotic drugs, Risperidone, which had recently come onto the market. As I recall, she was admitted on a Thursday, preliminary tests were done on a Friday and Risperidone cautiously introduced prior to the weekend. By the following Tuesday I was involved on the 'teaching ward round', with a dozen or so students in train. I had explained the circumstances of the story leading to her admission and pointed out the specific features of Lewy Body dementia. When I asked how she was, and what was happening to the gnomes, she said that they had now 'packed up and gone home'. The tale was further elucidated, revealing that upon her admission, the two families of gnomes had accompanied her and set up camp in alternate corners of her side-room. As the Risperidone took effect, the gnomes who had come on holiday with their suitcases, started literally to pack their bags and one by one, disappeared, waving her a cheery goodbye. By the Wednesday, she was gnome-free and was able to return home.

This book has had a long gestation and was originally inspired in my early twenties, by flicking through a book, entitled 'Brewers Dictionary of Phrase and Fable', which had been published in 1870 in a large second-hand book store. Its author, The Reverend Dr Ebenezer Brewer, had jotted down useful scraps of knowledge on odd bits of paper through much of his literate life and the book was the apotheosis of these thoughts. In parts, the book was quite incoherent, littered with random bits of history, anecdotes and comments. I thought it was great and started my own such collection from which is drawn much of my book.

This book, again, contrary to the title, is not designed to be 'wise'. It is in fact a collection of anecdotes and observations, drawn from the fields of student life, general medicine, geriatric medicine, domiciliary visiting and time spent on exercise with the Territorial Army. Any wisdom is probably contained within the sections on medico-legal medicine.

It is not intended to be an autobiography. However, it begins as such simply because in order to set the scene chronologically, there are certain autobiographical elements. To protect the 'guilty' from embarrassment, pseudonyms have been used, but real names have been used for those who have inspired me.

Advice has been plentiful and opinions as to how to do it, liberally expressed. Much of this has been genuinely appreciated. However, opinions are like 'arseholes', everyone has one and everyone thinks that everybody else's stinks.

Mark Twain said writing is easy; all you have to do is to cross out the wrong words. I have also drawn from the example of James Herriot, who wrote the famous series about veterinary practice. I am told that many of the stories in his books never actually happened to him but were either from elsewhere, apocryphal or fictional. My recollections may be similar – that is for the reader to fathom. However, there are some stories, so bizarre, that quite frankly you could not make them up.

The works of Jerome K Jerome have given me much amusement over the years and have provided me with a guide as to the ways and means of inserting various asides to educate and inform the reader as random thoughts crop up.

I am not yet in my anecdotage: apparently, this is what happens when you get old and dotty and sit around telling people stories about the 'good old days' all the time. There are, however, some useful musings and random use of anagrams, which I hope the reader will find entertaining.

For many of my newspaper cuttings and jottings, collected over many years, the source is unknown, though I can thank the Daily and Sunday Telegraph for having supplied oddities and their letter page is always inspiring. My copy of The Chronicle of the 20th Century has allowed me to check the timings of historic events and the numerous reliable sources available on the internet, particularly Wikipedia have allowed me to "flesh out" some issues. I shall remember my grammar and in particular, I shall try to carefully avoid the split infinitive. The spell-check should sort out my spelling and if neither the spell-checker nor I can spell Armageddon, it is not the end of the world.

For their inspiration, I would like to thank the following:- Paige Turner; Carrie Oakey: Anna Sasin; Barry Cade; Paul Bearer; Emma Rage; Anna Prentice; Isaac Hunt; Emma Royds and Chris Cross. Theresa Green has pointed out the blindingly obvious and Barb Dwyer has kept me on the right track for the military section.

Enjoy!

CHAPTER ONE

The Beginning

Life is a sexually transmitted condition with 100% mortality.

The question here is at what point does the beginning start? I arrived in the world, at Stepping Hill Hospital in Stockport, on the 30th December, 1952, following a prolonged and difficult natural labour, assisted, allegedly, by midwives Breda and Bertha. Stepping Hill Hospital was, and still is, a fine institution despite the local wags often repeating the phrase "step in ill, step out dead", perhaps because the short road from the A6 to the main entrance is unfortunately flanked on either side by two funeral parlours. Back to my arrival. I have rarely met any woman who claims to have had an easy labour. Midwifery must be quite interesting – meeting new people most days. According to my Chronical of the Twentieth Century, nothing much else happened on that day.

I did not choose my parents, they were chosen for me, by fate.

By way of background, my father was born in the provincial town of Neath in South Wales, in 1919. He had a reasonably comfortable, middle class upbringing, entering Neath Grammar School at the age of eleven. Whilst there, he excelled academically and was apparently a good team sportsman in both cricket and rugby. He went up to Swansea University to read Humanities in the autumn of 1938 and was destined for an academic career. The storm clouds of war were, however, gathering over Europe, and by April 1939 the Government was planning to introduce conscription, which was actioned and gathered pace during May 1939. In order to minimise disruption to his university studies, my father went for preliminary military training in the summer of 1939, thinking he could get it over with during the long vacation. Having received some training when war broke out, he was one of the first to be conscripted. He underwent further training at Catterick and eventually, following aptitude testing etc., was transferred to the Royal Signals Corps, in which he spent the rest of the war rising to the rank of Sergeant (he reckoned that Staff Sergeants, abbreviated to S. Sergeants were the epitome of greatness – a comment lost on me for many years). He claimed never to have fired his rifle in anger but was involved in two major retreats. His military section was attached to Headquarters, somewhere well to the south of Dunkirk and he was in France for some two weeks following the last operations to evacuate troops from Dunkirk, which ceased on the 4th June 1940.

There was an attempt to gather the 'ragtag and bobtail' personnel under the command of the French General Weygand, but this was not successful. Ultimately my father, along with his entire section and numerous stragglers, eventually left France around the middle of June, on the deck of a tramp steamer which left La Rochelle shortly after the ship Lancastria had been sunk on the 17th June 1940. He arrived at an undisclosed South Wales port, filthy dirty, bearded, hungry, but grateful to be alive. The troops were disembarked, rounded up into units and dispatched hither and thither. He recalled Polish troops being mustered and put on a sealed train and sent, non-stop, to Scotland. At that time there was a fear of fifth Columnists and it was thought that some could be concealed within their ranks and for a time and until vetted they were stationed as far away from London, as possible. {The term fifth Columnist, meaning traitor/ spy/ enemy originated in the Spanish civil war some years earlier, when General Franco, who had four columns of regular troops, was aided by sympathetic civilians – the fifth column – behind the lines as he advanced across Spain} My father was given a seventy-two hour pass and as he lived relatively locally, was told to 'clear off home' and report back for duty when it expired. Meanwhile, his mother had received a telegram from Her Majesty's Government, informing her that he was 'missing and presumed dead'. When he arrived at his mother's door, in the pitch dark, still filthy dirty, bearded and carrying his rifle with a clip of 5 rounds, he banged on the door but was initially refused entry, as his mother, who did not recognise him, suspected he was a tramp, up to no good.

Eventually, having been fed and cleaned up, he re-joined his unit and in due course, he and his section found themselves on a troop ship, heading north. The fact that he had been issued with thermal underclothes suggested to him that they might be heading towards

Norway, though this was never disclosed and that campaign was in any event short-lived. In fact, the weather began to turn progressively warmer and they found themselves off the coast of Africa (where he swapped his thermal undies for bananas with the locals) and eventually told they were heading for Singapore. However, by the end of 1941, the Japanese had set their sights on the Malay Peninsular and Singapore and his ship turned off to Java landing him on the north of the island. {Those Japanese ambitions were a delayed and unintended consequence of British diplomacy in WW1. When Germany threatened global war against the British Empire using battle cruisers based in Chinese ports, we asked our then ally, Japan, to attack them and to invade that part of China – thus encouraging Japanese expansion into the Pacific which led ultimately to the infamy of Pearl Harbour} Again, his section was attached to Headquarters but after the final surrender of Singapore in the middle of February 1942 Java was invaded. His second retreat involved the frantic crossing of Java to the southern port of Cilacap, gathering up mostly Dutch rubber planters and their wives and children en-route with the Japanese in hot pursuit. Their journey was dangerously slowed by the Dutch insisting on bringing all their possessions with them (their excess baggage was eventually dumped into the dock at Cilacap to speed up the escape). Dad reckoned that his most terrifying moment was in a forest at dead of night, knowing the Japanese were close by and hearing the voice of an Officer order "fix bayonets" He once again found himself on a troop ship, dodging Japanese war ships and submarines, before eventually arriving in Colombo, just in time for the Japanese bombing of the city on the 5th April 1942. He recalled spending days, along with other troops, hauling bodies out of the docks and was rewarded with double rations for his pains. Ceylon (now Sri Lanka) prepared for a Japanese invasion, which fortunately never came. My father spent the rest of the war there dealing with the cypher machines. He had a local batman to attend to his needs and was provided with a metal bed. It had been standard practise to stand the feet of the bed in dishes of water to discourage climbing insects – however those dishes could easily become breeding grounds for mosquitos so risking malaria – but use of paraffin instead worked despite the health and safety aspects. Eventually he returned to the UK in late 1945 and was based in Cardiff, preparing for his demob. He had had enough of troop ships but did admit that triremes might be the merriest of them!

My mother, born in 1921, hailed from the small village of Tumble in Carmarthenshire. It was mostly a rural idyll, until rich seams of anthracite were discovered in the late nineteenth Century and a large mine built at the lower part of the village. This attracted many incomers seeking employment but essentially, the language of the village was Welsh and farming was a major occupation. Her father, a carpenter, had built a substantial house with a large vegetable plot. As was common, they kept a pig fed on food waste and chickens for eggs. The pig was slaughtered in the autumn and as is well known, the only part of a pig which can't be consumed is the squeal. Despite the depression, my mother had a reasonably comfortable upbringing, with no real food shortage. However, there was a lot of sickness at home and her father died in 1938 from tuberculosis. A sister had succumbed to what was colloquially called 'sleepy sickness' (encephalitis lethargica) and another sister succumbed to post encephalitic Parkinson's disease after the birth of a daughter. There was no effective treatment and she died in the 1950s. {These conditions may have been a delayed consequence of the "Spanish Flu" which was a worldwide pandemic during 1918-1919 and killed at least 50 million. There is evidence that the death rate was higher in those who were treated with aspirin. This flu virus was probably a new and highly virulent strain of the H1N1 type. Such strains have emerged periodically over recorded history, including the swine and bird flu of the 21st Century – best treated with oinkment to avoid aporkalypse – (when there was an outbreak in medieval renaissance Italy the cause was unknown but thought to have been from astrological influence – the "influenza" – hence the name). The virus seems to originate in birds and mutate in the presence of pigs. The close proximity of pigs, birds and people is not to be recommended. It got the name because Spain, not being involved in WW1, was one of the few countries to openly report it in the press. In fact it almost certainly originated in Haskell County, Kansas, USA where US servicemen at an army base, in close proximity to pigs and birds on local farms, were being trained prior to being shipped to the trenches}

Mum recalls speaking only Welsh at home but the language in school was English. Pupils were caned if heard speaking Welsh within the school grounds. The philosophy at the time was that use of the English medium was the root to success and school was the only environment in which it could be learnt.

My mother always claimed that she was clever but denied education beyond the school leaving age of thirteen, simply because her parents chose to pay – it was only free up to the age of 13 – to educate her brothers, rather than her. When she left school, she was destined to remain at home, assisting her mother with the significant household chores, before eventually, presumably getting married and running her own household. She rebelled against this and eventually trained as a dressmaker, having been taken on as an apprentice by a successful dressmaker, living locally. She reckoned the war provided the opportunity to escape the village.

When war was declared and before the call-up of young single women was introduced, her skill as a dressmaker was in great demand, for making parachutes. She found employment in a parachute factory near Cardiff docks, having arranged to stay with her cousin, William Rees and his wife. William Rees (my uncle Billy) was then a Detective Inspector in Cardiff Constabulary. (as an aside in later years Uncle Billy was an avid attender at family funeral events, which he always described as real fun and referring to the mother-in-law as Hitler woman – also lost on me for many years). (Whilst on the subject of funerals, I am reminded of a man whose frequent attendance at random funerals, on an almost daily basis was noticed by undertakers. He was dressed appropriately and always paid his respects to the bereaved. He was nicknamed the 'grim eater' as he was able to eat and drink for free for many months before he was rumbled). In due course, DI Rees was promoted and left Cardiff and my mother found lodgings elsewhere. She loved Cardiff for the freedom it gave her, despite having to endure the blitz. At some point, she acquired a large roll of parachute silk and circumvented clothes rationing by using it to make underwear – the remnant of that roll was still in their house when it was cleared in 2010.

In any event, my to-be parents were both stationed in Cardiff when they met. Fate determined that when my mother boarded a bus to return home for a visit to her parents, the only vacant seat on the bus was next to my father who was still in uniform. They obviously clicked because he pursued her with great ardour thereafter and they duly married in 1947.

Meanwhile, my father had taken advantage of a scheme to train returning servicemen with good academic qualifications as school teachers, on a shortened course. He never finished his degree.

Jobs in south Wales were scarce and depended more on 'who you knew', than what you knew. There were, however, vacancies in the north of England. Fate was such that Uncle Billy had been appointed as Chief Constable in Stockport and had purchased a fairly substantial house. My parents found lodgings there temporarily and my father employment in teaching. Pending my arrival and notwithstanding a number of miscarriages, my mother had trained as a children's nurse and worked for a time at a nursery, attached to a large cotton mill, owned by Uncle Billy's neighbour.

In the late 1940s and early 1950s there was a significant shortage of housing. Not only had many homes been destroyed by bombing but large numbers of returning servicemen, having had their lives on-hold during the war, were eager to marry and set up homes of their own. It so happened that a local and respected landlord committed some minor traffic offence, which attracted the attention of the police. Uncle Billy dealt with this himself, the upshot of which was that my parents were offered first refusal on a house to rent and no police action was taken on the landlord.

The Early Years

I was part of the baby boomer generation; there were children everywhere. Few mothers worked and my recollections were of a fairly carefree existence. However, the 1950s were dangerous times. There was a polio epidemic and the SALK and SABIN vaccines were yet to be developed. {This disease was a "crippler" rather than a killer. The virus was spread in people by the faecal-oral route and many children, especially if exposed to poor sanitation, met the less virulent strains naturally and acquired some form of natural immunity. Middle class children with better hygiene at home were less likely to have acquired immunity. Epidemics occurred when a virulent strain appeared. They were mostly in the summer months (cold weather killed it off). Minor illness amounting to no more than a few days of low grade fever, headache, malaise and vomiting was the commonest manifestation. The rarer major illness resulted in flaccid limb paralysis as the virus attacked the spinal cord. Swallowing and breathing problems occurred if the brain stem centres were attacked. With rest and good nursing care most recovered but were left with degrees of wasting and weakness to the muscle groups affected. Some required callipers to walk but most regained independence. Fifty-sixty years after the 1950's epidemic we are now seeing post-polio syndrome due to age related muscle wasting having a more profound effect on those areas previously weakened. (President F. D Roosevelt who had childhood polio but could stand and walk early in his term of office became wheelchair-bound later}

All children, if they were lucky, got their German measles, measles, mumps chickenpox and whooping cough, before they started school. In fact, to encourage this, healthy children were often paraded in front of those diseased at "spot parties", in order to acquire conditions as soon as possible. Measles was indeed misery and the serious complication of brain-damaging pansclerosing encephalitis and death could occur. Whooping cough was easily recognisable by the characteristic coughing of people that went on for many months. {A traditional "cure" for whooping cough was the drinking of mare's milk. In the 1920s-1930s when milk was delivered door-to-door in open churns, pulled by a horse and trap and ladled out to you in your jug by the road-side, such mare's milk could be obtained, at cost, if the horse pulling the milk float was a lactating mare. She would be milked by hand in the gutter}.

The NHS had been established and had removed much of the fear of penury from disease. Free dental care was available and this had ended the practice of brides having their teeth removed prophylactically after their wedding, to avoid the expensive costs of pre-NHS dentistry, should things go wrong. {Some dental fixative creams contain Zinc which can be absorbed. We need small amounts of Zinc and Copper in our diets to optimise health and a sensible diet provides them naturally. However, they are absorbed by a common route and too much Zinc can overload the pathway and lead to Copper deficiency. Whilst rare, I have seen this once, causing weird neurological weakness – Copper deficiency causes "the staggers" in cattle but probably not anything denture related!}

Smoking was prevalent. Everyone smoked, pregnant women smoked, even non-smokers smoked by puffing on a cigarette, just to fit in. You could smoke everywhere, except on the lower deck of a double decker bus. No one seemed to smoke in Church, presumably out of respect or maybe wariness that the fire and brimstone in the sermons would spoil the taste. The Doctor smoked, the Dentist smoked; they smoked in their surgeries; patients smoked in the waiting rooms, patients would smoke in their hospital beds. Even children got in on the act. There were sweet cigarettes, bought in packs of ten – a small stick of candy, with red at one end. Chocolate cigarettes and cigars were common stocking-fillers at Xmas. For the sophisticated child, you could buy imitation cigarettes. These were hollow tubes of paper, with a red foil end. The tube contained fine-grade talcum powder and the foil tip was perforated. By blowing into the tube, you could create the illusion of smoke. For convenience, cigarettes were sold in packs of five, ten, twenty and tins of fifty. The novice school boy smoker could usually persuade a tobacconist to sell single cigarettes (Loosies) and a hand full of matches to go with it. If the shops were shut, vending machines were on street corners. If you had a minor accident, you were given a cigarette to steady the nerves; if you were upset, you were given a cigarette and perhaps a glass of brandy. {Nicotine interferes with the conversion of DOPA to catecholamines and reduces anxiety and panic}. If you had a weak chest, strong cigarettes were advised to toughen the lungs. In short, smoking was a normal and completely unremarkable activity. There was no antismoking Lobby and the handful of people who did object were considered to be cranks – this may have had something to do with the fact that the recently defeated and dead Adolph Hitler had been a rabid antismoker. The link between smoking and lung cancer was not properly established until 1954 and denied by many for years thereafter!

I think my parents, along with many, struggled in the early 50s. Money was in short supply and rationing of certain items continued for a year or two after my birth. No one ate on the streets, obesity was very rare and the rare plump kids acquired the nickname "fatty". There were no fast-food outlets apart from Fish and Chip shops – which surprisingly sold just that! The source of heat in most houses came from coal fires, which had a back-boiler to provide hot water. If chimneys were not regularly swept, soot accumulated therein and could catch fire. We children were always amused at seeing flames shooting from the chimney pots on the roof. Normally, only one room in the house was heated and on cold winter days, people huddled around the fire, toasting their fronts, whilst freezing their backs. Ladies with bare legs, sitting close to the fire, would acquire a mottled permanent appearance to their legs – erythema ab igne, from the skin damage caused by a combination of heat and flame. From the distribution, you could make an educated guess as to which side of the fireplace they preferred to sit. Bedrooms were freezing and it was normal to wake up on a cold winter's day, to find that the condensation on the windows from breath had frozen solid, such that there was more frost on the inside of the window, than on the outside.

On the wider stage, the 1950s were politically dangerous. The Cold War was at its peak. I would regularly see Vulcan bombers flying over our house, allegedly fully primed with nuclear weapons (these have long been mothballed but one was re-commissioned and used during the Falkland conflict of 1982). The Korean War and Suez crisis occurred during my early childhood and my father, although long out of the Army, was on a reserve list and for a while feared being recalled. My early schooling was enjoyable but unremarkable and as an only child, until my brother appeared on the scene in 1960, I led a fairly happy, carefree existence. I was blissfully unaware of the dangers of the world and my first awareness of any threat, came from reading about the Moors Murders in the paper. The reading about the "Profumo Scandal", armed with a dictionary, considerably advanced my education! During the early 60s, my education focused upon the absolute necessity of passing the 11+ examination. This examination, taken at the age of eleven, was a 'make or break' situation for the future. If you passed (yes, words like 'pass' and 'fail' were used routinely), you got a place in a grammar school and could be reasonably assured of a decent education. If you were male and had a borderline pass, you might be offered a place in a technical school but for the 75%-80% of people who failed, they were destined to receive a fairly mediocre education at a secondary modern school. I was fortunate in passing the 11+ and entered Stockport School in the September of 1964.

The End of the Beginning

Arriving in the 'big' school was a shock. On day one, a hundred and fifty others (boys only) also started, often being bused in from far flung suburbs of the town. I was lucky; it was within walking distance for me. One hundred and fifty students were divided into five forms and in the first year, taught everything. I loathed art and music but gradually, was able to drop the subjects I disliked, in order to focus on those that would suit my aim. I had realised by the age of 14 that I wished to do medicine and applied myself to my studies. I recall a comment from my early years 'it's your attitude not your aptitude that affects your altitude'. I have a collection of school reports and comments therein (not all mine), which are worth sharing:

Report for Woodwork: "Give him the job and he will finish the tools"

Geography: "Does well to find his way back home each day"

Music: "Live wire, low voltage"

Latin: "He has given me a new definition of the word stoicism – he grins and I bear it"

French: "By the time he has mastered French, he will be too old to cross the Channel"

English: "The improvement in his handwriting has revealed his inability to spell"

Woodwork (again): "When the workers of the world unite, it will be presumptuous of Geoffrey to include himself in their number"

Art: "Geoffrey attended the lessons"

Art (again): "I am sorry to have to tell you that he is doing his best"

Religious Education: "This boy does not need a scripture teacher, he needs a missionary"

After 'O' Levels taken at sixteen, the majority of my entry cohort left school. The only point of staying on to do 'A' Levels was to go to University – only some 5% of 18 year olds did. Roughly thirty of us (20% of the original entry) entered the Lower Sixth, with varying aims and knuckled down to a fairly intense, two years of study to reap the appropriate glistening prize. Not all Medical Schools interviewed and I was accepted on the basis of my academic track record, with the requirement that I achieved at least three grade 'Cs'. In fact, I got an 'A' in biology, 'B' in chemistry and a 'C' in physics.

In retrospect, I was a relatively conscientious individual and got up to relatively few pranks; I was also always conscious of the Eleventh Commandment "Thou Shalt Not Be Found Out".

Of the mischief to which I am prepared to admit, knowledge of chemistry assisted.

Some protractors were made of a particular type of rigid plastic which we would break up into smaller pieces. If wrapped tightly in foil and ignited, large amounts of sweet-smelling white smoke would result. The rule of thumb was that just over half a protractor's worth of plastic in 4 pieces treated this way and spread about could make a form room unusable for an hour.

We had our own version of "Darts" played if unsupervised between lessons and at break. Take one standard darning needle and some lead foil. Fold the foil tightly around the needle 1cm from the point and solder firmly in place. Thread the eye with about a foot of strong fishing line. Stand at the back of the form room and whirl it about one's head to gather momentum before releasing in the general direction of the blackboard. The lead added sufficient weight for these missiles to easily travel the distance and embed themselves up to the foil ring.

I recall making the highly explosive nitrogen triiodide, by dissolving iodine crystals in concentrated ammonia. This was perfectly stable when moist and could be flicked on the floor with a brush, brushed onto door handles and painted onto benches, chairs and toilet seats. Once it was dry, it was highly unstable and the least contact would cause a reassuringly loud crack. In the small quantities used, it was not at all dangerous, just a bit of fun.

The run up to Bonfire night provided a ready source of gunpowder, allowing potentially extremely dangerous activities to occur. At a simple level, wrapping a banger with clay dug from the garden, lighting it and throwing it would make a fairly impressive grenade. Small cannons could be made from suitable cast-off tubes, fired using the gunpowder, the usual missile being a glass marble.

Living within easy reach of the Peak District, my friends and I would regularly take the bus to Hayfield and hike over Kinder Scout. Cycling to Lyme Park took only half an hour uphill but freewheeling back was much faster and in retrospect quite dangerous as that road was very busy. We once went as far as the Cat and Fiddle pub on the A537 between Macclesfield and Buxton, mainly for the pleasure of freewheeling back. That pub is the second highest inn in England and we managed to get served (at 15yrs of age) with half pints of beer at the cost of, I think, 11d each – now 5p {The origin of the pub's name is uncertain perhaps from Le Chat Fidele (faithful cat) or Catherine et Fidele (Catherine of Aragon is faithful). Decimalisation of the British coinage was introduced in February 1971 such that there were 100p to the pound instead of the previous twenty shillings each of 12d.}

From 1954 the family home had been 262, Dialstone lane – a short walk from both Stepping Hill Hospital and school. I had a Saturday job in a greengrocer's shop on the A6 in nearby Great Moor and well remember the initial confusion when decimalisation came in. {Great Moor was and is an unremarkable small suburban area of small shops but historically has a claim to fame as the place where the last man in England (James Dean) was gibbeted – I presume that his execution was an exit on cue! Gibbeting usually meant suspending a corpse in public until it finally rotted away or was eaten by crows. The word gibbet also means a scaffold for execution – the most famous and unusual one being in Halifax which was effectively a Guillotine (200+ years ahead of the French) constructed from an executioner's axe set in a block of wood and dropped in a frame and in use roughly from 1541-1650}. Stockport itself is famous for hat manufacturing and as the source of the river Mersey.

The all-male environment of Stockport School was fairly daunting at 11. Masters wore academic gowns and corporal punishment was dished out fairly freely to the naughty squad (if caught). During the autumn of 1966 our form room developed a growing stench of rotting fish which varied according to the time of day – worse in the late afternoon and with the benefit of hindsight progressively earlier in the afternoon as Xmas approached. Mornings were generally not too bad. A prank was suspected. Desks and lockers were searched, dire threats made and the likely suspects interviewed in depth but to no avail. It continued. The lifting of the floorboards over the Xmas Holidays failed to elucidate the cause. The smell gradually lessened in the spring and vanished in the summer only to return with a vengeance the following late autumn with the same pattern. It was not a prank – one of the ancient plastic (made of casein-formaldehyde we found out later) ceiling lampshades had slipped such that it was resting directly on the light bulb and was decomposing from heat when the lights were on, releasing the appalling stink.

Teaching was generally of high standard and not as tightly restricted to the curriculum as is now the case. The last few days of each term afforded opportunities for the masters to teach life skills and impart more light-hearted knowledge often drawn from very wide and varied life experiences from time spent in the real world before they took up teaching. (It wouldn't have happened like this had girls been present). I recall the following:-

Examples of how to use the F*** word correctly and imaginably.

Following some bother, the German commandant of a POW camp addressed paraded British troops in English with the words "You think we Germans know F*** nothing" he told them "but in fact" he continued with growing confidence "we know F*** all" Accompanied by much mirth and collapse of parade ground discipline.

When a British tank broke down for the umpteenth time on active service, the exasperated sergeant having poked about in the engine for a while, flung down his spanner exclaiming "The f***ing, F***er has f***ing well F***ed it's f***ing self, sir".

Religion:

Israeli cheeses are a delicacy, especially cheeses of Nazareth.

Rich saints are Christians.

We know that Moses wore a wig because only sometimes he was seen with Aaron.

Adam blamed Eve; Eve blamed the snake because he didn't have a leg to stand on.

Ladies who wished to join the Mother's Union were invited to see the Vicar after services.

Trade unionists 23rd Psalm:

The Union is my shepherd.

I shall not work.

It maketh me to lie down on the job.

It leadeth me beside still factories.

It restoreth my insurance benefits.

Yea tho' I walk through the shadow of decreased productivity.

I will fear no recrimination for the union is with me.

Its restrictive practises and shop stewards, they comfort me.

It prepareth a works committee for me in the presence of my employers.

It annointeth my hand with pay rises.

My bank balance runneth over.

Surely never-never payments and union dues shall follow me all the days of my life.

And I shall dwell in the Council Flats for ever.

Language;

Palindromes – Was it Eliot's toilet I saw?

Sex at noon taxes.

A man, a plan, a canal: Panama.

Doc, note. I dissent. A fast never prevents a fatness. I diet on cod.

Words which have no rhyming words in English include silver, purple, orange, cusp, bilge, bulb, scarce, month, warmth, film and spoilt.

The Greek sentence – Ouk elabon polin, alla gar elpis ephe kaka (they did not take the city as they hadn't any real chance) if read with a French accent becomes –

Ou qu'est la bonne Pauline? A la gare elle pisse et fait caca which translates as

Where is good Pauline? At the station, she pees and shits.

SPAM stands for Shit Posing as Meat.

That going like Billio comes from the preacher Joseph Billio who gave his sermons with great Gusto.

Fanny Adams was an 8-year-old girl, butchered to death in a Kent hop field in 1867. Her name was used by troops to describe army issue canned mutton chops.

Testiculation is the art of using flamboyant gestures whilst talking a load of old bollocks.

The British Empire:

We learnt of exotic characters. The Fakir of Ipi who would feed his enemies to crocodiles; the Wali of Swat (just because of his name) and a northern Nigerian tribal chieftain by the name of the Tigwe of Vwuip who as late as 1960 had to be arrested having eaten the local tax inspector. Bishop Savage who headed the Diocese of Zululand and Swaziland liked to introduce himself as "Savage of Zululand".

Final School leaving advice "When in doubt, do the decent thing".

CHAPTER TWO

The Pre-Clinical Years

Come late September 1971, I arrived in Cardiff, and booked into the University Hall of Residence in Cyncoed. Why Cardiff? Well, firstly it was a pleasant city, then there were family connections and the Welsh National School of Medicine had an excellent reputation. It was sufficiently far from home for me to get up to mischief unobserved and frequent returns home were not expected. The apron strings had been cut! Extended family, however, were within sufficiently close distance for a day's visit if I fancied, and Uncle Billy and his wife had retired and moved to nearby Penarth. So, in preparation for this, I had completed my UCCA form (the forerunner of the UCAS) in the autumn of 1970, and in due course, was offered a place dependent upon adequate 'A' Levels. I did visit one or two other places on designated open days, but not Cardiff. Many of my contemporaries thought it a great skive to swan off courtesy of a day off school, to have a look round and feel the ambience of "uni". I remember a bunch going on a train up to Newcastle. I think they numbered about five in total but upon arrival back at Stockport Station, where some of the fathers had arranged to meet them, one of their number was missing. His father immediately noticed his absence. After some evasive answers, it turned out that the little darling had got himself hopelessly drunk on the train and his so-called mates had abandoned him on the platform of Durham Station. So much for pure ales giving pleasure! Few rites of passage in these isles of ours are unaccompanied by a bottle. His father was particularly hopping mad that his mates had not stuck with him (as an aside, a similar episode later occurred to Euan one of the sons of Tony Blair, when his father was Prime Minister). As parents, most of us have been there! These irresponsible reckless acts seem to be a male characteristic, borne of the fact that young men's brains don't fully wire until their mid-twenties. In any event, lots of telephone calls to the Station Master at Durham, followed by phone calls to local hospitals and police stations, established that indeed, they had a young man who fitted the description, locked up in a cell for being drunk and disorderly. The concerned father dropped one of the 'mates' at home with some disgust, and hared off in the car to Durham. Now this man was a mature individual, he had seen action in the Second World War, he knew what suffering was like, he knew what squalor was like; he was a man of the world, yet, when he saw the sight before him, he was visibly shocked. His son had vomited numerous times, he had become doubly incontinent, his trousers were ripped, his shirt was torn and he had been unceremoniously dumped in the cell and was curled up on the floor unconscious. There had been no attempt whatsoever to clean him up. I am not party to what negotiations occurred in the 'Nick' but the upshot was that he was released into his father's custody, wrapped in an old blanket, bundled into the back of the car (windows open of course) and driven home. The incident was never mentioned again.

In the summer of 1971, I spent a long period in Brittany, mostly based around an exchange visit to Nantes. The weather was glorious and I had sufficient knowledge of the French language to get about. Some innocent (well sort of innocent) fumbling, on my part, in the skimpy underwear of a willing mademoiselle behind some bushes on a park bench attracted the attention of someone I believed to be the uniformed park-keeper – the "parky". When I attempted to give him short-shrift in my rudest French he drew his pistol, at which point I realised that he probably was not a mere 'parky'. I had no ID and few francs on my person and was over 18. Technically by those criteria and according to the law of the land I was a vagrant and arrested as such. Handcuffs followed, a black Maria arrived to provide transport and la belle mademoiselle who had ID and francs "vamoosed" – I learned later from the wise men of the world that women, along with cats and monkeys, cannot be trusted. The aftermath of the Algerian war of independence with terrorist attacks by the OAS resentful that De Gaulle had eventually abandoned that country and the "pied noir" within, had heightened the security at French police stations and such tight security was still in evidence years later. Those bastions of power bore little resemblance to "Dock Green". Entrances had armed guards and there was no friendly sergeant behind the desk. After a night in the cells I was eventually vouched for and released. I am not sure if I have a French criminal record or not! I was not deported and my passport received no obvious stamp indicating my vagrancy status, though for some years my pulse quickened at French passport controls. I received the results of my 'A' Levels, sent on an old fashioned tele-printer by one of my teachers from school; I needed to do nothing except celebrate, with plenty of cheap French wine and plan my future. {France is a lovely country but with some odd laws. Since 1959 it has been legal to marry a dead person provided you can prove that the marriage was already planned – some 20 are approved by the President annually – presumably consummation is unnecessary as that would be dead boring. They say by contrast that incest is only relatively so}.

University Hall, Cardiff was an old fashioned Hall of Residence. My room was basic and comfortable. There was a bed, a chair, a desk, an easy-chair, a bookshelf and a wardrobe. There were no en-suite facilities but there was a communal bathroom down the corridor and a very small kitchenette, with a Baby-Belling stove, sufficient to make toast and heat up a pan of whatever. Lydia cleaned the communal areas daily and the rooms weekly. Catering, however, was all-in. A substantial cooked breakfast was available all mornings, but no lunch. In the evenings, there were two sittings. There was an early sitting at about 5.30 pm, of a buffet nature or a later sitting at 7.30 pm, which was more formal, with waitresses serving at the table. I and most of my friends preferred to eat early and return to our rooms to study, until about 8.30 pm and then regroup in the bar/recreation lounge, for a few drinks. I excelled at football – well actually table football – with my prowess improving progressively with the passage of time and the consumption of beer at the princely price of 15p/pint. {I have it on good authority that the patron saint of football referees is St. Off} My friend Gwynfor (reading maths) and I made a formidable premier league duo. Through him I got to know and associate with a disreputable crowd of mining/mineral exploitation students which led to me acquiring the unjustified (in my eyes) soubriquet as being "the mad medic". Talk about giving a dog a bad name – more later!

Gwynfor was on the bar committee. As such he had to take turns in charge of the bar. At busy periods, anyone could help out in return for free drinks. Once weekly the beer pipes had to be cleaned – normally on a Sunday afternoon. I would sometimes help him out if it was his turn. On one such day, when the beer was obviously "off tap" we turned to the spirit optics for libation and fell asleep in mid-task. He blamed me for leading him astray! Some of the mining/mineral exploitation students were keen potholers and one day I tagged along. Wearing the gear including a miner's helmet and light, I abseiled underground and walked along a narrow shelf above a yawning chasm, supporting myself with hands touching the wall on the other side of the drop. The problem was that the shelf narrowed as the chasm widened such that at one point I was almost horizontal before we turned off into a passage. Narrow crawls followed culminating in a "sump". This is like going through the U-bend of the toilet {Some idiot my father knew back in Stockport was known behind his back as Harpic because he was allegedly clean round the bend – having done this, risking life and limb. I thought I deserved that title}. After all day underground, I was glad to see daylight.

The Hall of Residence was a short walk from Roath Park with its boating lake and some half hour's brisk walk from the University centre. Every morning, a large crocodile of students would make that journey on foot. Fresher's week, as now, was a round of queuing, collecting various passes, documents, (the all-important grant cheque) and investigating whether to join certain societies. I was not particularly sporty and avoided anything to do with politics, religion or general do-gooding. I was there purely to drink, study and womanise. As a parody of Julius Caesar with his "veni, vidi vici" many students tried to see, conquer and come. It is said that an intellectual is someone who has found something more interesting than sex. By that definition, I lacked the qualification to join their number.

My parents had taken a dim view about the various student unrest in universities in the 60s and I was mature enough to observe that studies were more important. Oft quoted at home was the example of some distant family member who, whilst at university, had joined the Communist Party in the 1930s, becoming a "card-carrying member". Politics was serious in those days, with extreme left and right wing factions vying for the attentions of 'bright' people attending university. Apparently, it was common practice for attractive and somewhat promiscuous young women to latch onto targets, getting them to sign up as party members. Fine – most of the time and indeed, during the War, Stalin was our ally and being a Communist, not necessarily harmful. However, with the advent of the Cold War, anyone who had extreme left wing sympathies and was in a position of power paid the price. This was particularly so in the USA (McCarthyism) but also occurred to a certain extent in ordinary UK provincial town life – old sins cast long shadows.

My mother's advice was to join the local church, where I might meet a "nice type of girl". Quelle Horreur! What eighteen-year-old male, away from home, with his own lockable room and a bed, wants to meet a nice type of girl? Well, I did want to meet a nice type of girl but not necessarily the sort that my mother would think that I ought to meet (my wife does not like me telling this tale). Well, I think enough said, as a gentleman should not discuss these matters.

The course was fairly traditional and for the first two years, there was no patient contact whatsoever. We were basically busy 9-5, five days a week, on the main University campus in the city centre studying anatomy, (the basic structure of the body), physiology (how it worked) and biochemistry. Some very basic sociology and psychology was also thrown in.

Anatomy was learnt partly from books – essential facts – the clitoris with 8,000 nerve endings per square inch has double the number in the glans penis – no wonder those organs make groans! As some previous owner had scribbled in the margin of my anatomy book, the largest vein in the vagina is the dorsal vein of the penis! Mostly anatomy was learnt from dissecting a human cadaver donated to science under the guidance of trainee surgeons who were preparing for the surgical fellowship exams by spending a year doing extra anatomy. It was a fantastic and humbling experience to go on a voyage of discovery through the human body. The dissecting manuals were our map and Sat-Nav.

Without these selfless acts of donation such experiences would have been impossible. The numbered bodies were respected and all the pieces removed were returned to the appropriate identically numbered receptacle such that the complete remains could be cremated (apparently at the expense of the University) at the end of the year. Each cadaver lasted a year. A group of four first years dissected the whole body alternating during the week with four second years who concerned themselves with the much more complex head and neck anatomy. There were no "high jinks" with body parts. {I did however hear that at some time in the past, a keen student had taken an arm wrapped in brown paper home on the bus for further study. Unfortunately, some distraction (probably more likely a woman or cat than a monkey) caused him to leave it behind when he alighted. Aghast at the potential consequences of this harmless act, he confessed to a bus inspector and in due course was re-united with the arm in "lost property" A liberal tip ensured lack of career consequence. The corpse of Oliver Cromwell which had been embalmed was disinterred (along with the other signatories of the death warrant of Charles 1st) after the restoration of Charles 2nd and their heads placed in public view on poles for some twenty years. Cromwell's pole snapped in a storm in the 1680's and his head fell into the London streets. His face was still recognisable from the combination of embalming and weathering. It was found by an anti-royalist, kept as a relic and in due course sold on. After passing through the hands of various fairground showmen it was finally buried in 1960 in a secret spot in or near the chapel of his old Cambridge College (Sidney Sussex) to whose master the secret is revealed upon appointment. (Allegedly, as a baby, Oliver was scooped up by the family pet monkey and carried on to the roof – remember you can't trust a monkey). The skull of Ned Kelly went walkabout after being disinterred. The remains of Geronimo, the Apache leader who died as a POW in 1909, were allegedly dug up from his grave at Fort Still, Oklahoma, in 1918 by a trio including an ancestor of President Bush, and taken to Yale. They are said to remain in the custody of a secret "skull and bones" student society, whose "bones men" kiss his skull on initiation. At what point does a grave-robbing morph into archaeology?}

We had to learn all the muscles, the nerve supplies and the relationship between all the structures, to a standard that would have allowed us the anatomical knowledge to operate, if we had had the necessary surgical skills. All muscles attach to bones and to understand the relationships, we were encouraged to purchase a skeleton. To be more accurate, it was a half skeleton, containing one of everything of which you had two and all the bits of which you had one (apparently, these bones were sourced primarily from India, cleaned and processed in Cornwall as a winter industry when the fishing was slack, and packaged up and sold. They were real bones and the whole process was coordinated and regulated by some central-body). Obviously, these skeletons were second-hand but there was a small little side-line industry, whereby students would sell on their books and the already second-hand skeleton to the next generation, when they became superfluous to need after the second year. The proceeds went on clinical books and a decent stethoscope. The boxes in which skeletons came were fairly bulky and certainly far too bulky to transport home on the train, along with other possessions. At the end of my first year, a girl I knew, who had a flat in Cardiff, agreed to look after my skeleton. We had had a somewhat loose relationship but I thought that when I collected the skeleton, we might or might not resume where we had left off. In any event, that was not to be and I found myself walking home from her flat, at about 1 am, carrying my fairly substantial box. This attracted the attention of the local constabulary, who quite reasonably asked what some scruffy student was carrying in his arms. When I replied a skeleton, I got 'nicked' and found myself in a police station yet again, being asked awkward questions. I had no ID to prove that I was a student or indeed that I was a medical student with a perfectly legitimate reason to be carrying a skeleton around the streets. There didn't seem much that I could do at that time in the morning but by luck, a passing police surgeon had come in to sort out the drunks and I asked him to give me a mini-viva, asking the questions, which only a legitimate medical student could answer (I think he had forgotten a lot of his anatomy, because the questions he asked were so basic that I obviously knew more than him). In any event, I passed and got driven back to my Halls by the police. I thoroughly enjoyed anatomy and although I have used relatively little of the knowledge in my career, certain bits have stayed with me. We learned some complex bits using mnemonics. I recall "As she lay flat Oswald's penis slowly mounted" but am now clueless as to what it prompted me to remember. The phrase "The lingual nerve, it made a swerve around the hyoglossus. Said Wharton's duct, Well I'll be f***ed, this bugger's going to cross us" at least now makes some sense. My anatomy dissecting manuals were kept, mainly because the jottings in the margins made them unsaleable. Even now, after forty years, opening the pages gives the faint whiff of the preservative formalin, which was used on the cadavers. Smells arouse memories like nothing else. As I muse, I am reminded of a popular perfume of those days "Kiku" which, if I could find, might revive some long-forgotten but likely delightful memories.

Domestically, I had been well-trained when I left home. I was perfectly capable of cooking and keeping myself and my room clean and tidy and sorting out my washing and ironing in the mini-laundrette provided at the Hall of Residence site. Some were however poorly prepared. Stan Stillman had arrived in Halls from boarding school and lacked any basic skills. In the first few weeks of term, when the weather was fairly warm, the obnoxious aroma from a growing pile of dirty socks, heaped in the corner of his room, started to permeate the corridors. The cleaners refused to go in and the smell gradually became unbearable, even Stan himself realised there was a problem and hung the dirty socks out of his window on a piece of string (why he didn't actually get them washed, I will never know). The corridors then became smell-free but his neighbours were unable to open their own windows because of the stench. It was eventually solved by Wayne Scales taking matters in hand by unfurling the fire hose and hosing the offending socks off the window sill and freshening them up. Wayne was a dental student and as such, his need to know anatomy was limited to the head and neck. Most dental students purchased a skull. Wayne had a particularly splendid example, with the styloid processes still intact (these are fragile bits that are of little relevance and normally snap off in the hands of students). At some point, in the first weeks of student life, Wayne had pinched a flashing traffic cone and had dumped the orange case, being left with the light on a small stick. His skull sat upon it, with the light up the foramen magnum, such that when placed on his window sill, the flashing skull could be seen for some distance. It looked fairly impressive. He was also a fan of the then popular Tartan beer. In fact, his consumption of this had been heroic, such that by the end of the first term, he had created a mini colonnade from used cans sellotaped together. His bed had been turned into a four-poster, his wardrobe had been artistically framed in beer cans and there was a central pillar. At some point, someone down my corridor had acquired a shop mannequin, which was dressed and hung out of the window. From a distance, this looked like a suicide by hanging. We students knew what it was. However, Cyncoed was an affluent suburban area, the Hall of Residence having been built within the grounds of a very substantial house. Some interfering busy-body, who had spotted this from their bedroom window, had alerted the authorities, which resulted in the flashing blue lights of a police car and ambulance arrival onsite.

Ann Teak was not a student; she was an attractive local young nymphomaniac who had taken the practise of that condition to new heights. She was the "Martini Girl" of legend – anytime, anywhere, any place. Her modus operandi (so I have been told) was very effective. She would wander around the male corridors of University Hall in the evenings and randomly knock on doors with some seemingly innocent request. If she was invited in, she would head for the bed strip off and make it perfectly obvious why she was there. She was rarely refused. After the event, she would quietly leave to continue her perambulations. This must have gone on for months – no one had been saying anything – until over some drinks one lad let slip what had happened to him the previous evening. The scene which followed was reminiscent of the film "Spartacus" when large numbers claimed to be him. Ann had been at it most nights with at least 5 "scores" on some nights. Years later I heard that she had not aged well. She had become a master-baker and opened a small shop named "Crusty Bloomers" on the high street.

My introduction to basic statistics was most illuminating. It occurred in one of the early physiology lectures, given towards the end of Fresher's week. There were roughly one hundred in my entry year and unusually for the time, almost 50% were female. The law of large numbers allows certain predictions to be made. For the one hundred in our year, the following predictions (reasonably accurate as it turned out) were made:

i)   One of us would die before the course was over.

ii) One of us would go mad.

iii) Roughly 85 would become general practitioners.

iv) Two people would become consultant physicians.

v)   Two would become consultant surgeons.

vi) Three would fail the course.

vii) The remainder would find diverse niches in various specialisms.

Physiology itself was a fascinating subject and we performed certain experiments upon one another.

Biochemistry provided insight into the way in which the chemistry of the body worked at an intracellular level. The only compulsory 'A' Level for entry into medical school in my day was chemistry. Most people had also done physics and biology but there were some people who had not done biology beyond 'O' Level. It seemed to be those people who found biochemistry particularly hard to master. One useful fact I learned was that dietary fat influences the body fat – cooking oil gives more fluid fatty tissue whereas butter and dripping produces firmer body fat. In later years, I would hear old sex offenders lament that young female breasts had become less firm over the last 50 years! To move into clinical medicine from the third year onwards, the formidable second MB examination had to be passed at the end of the second year (First MB, which almost no one ever took, was apparently the equivalent of 'A' Levels, which some aspiring medical students, without school science could take as an entrance qualification to do medicine by spending an extra preliminary year at University). This examination required a detailed knowledge of all those three subjects. Fortunately, it all seemed to gel together in my mind and by the time I took it, I felt I had an excellent understanding of the whole workings of the human body and could relate the interplay between the anatomy, physiology and biochemistry perfectly. Unfortunately, some 10% of the year failed, with the opportunity to re-sit in the September. Stan Stillman, who had bucked up his domestic ideas since the firehose incident, unfortunately failed. He was unceremoniously collected by his parents and bundled off home for intense cramming. His father, a Doctor, meanwhile, had revised his own mostly forgotten anatomy, to a level whereby he could teach Stan. Stan passed and went on to have an illustrious career. Some four people failed and left the course completely but mostly transferred to other University degrees. During those first two years, the course was the three standard University terms, encompassing some thirty-six weeks. I along with others was able to enjoy a long summer vacation (with a holiday job) before return in the September to start our clinical studies. The job was at a local hotel assisting the in-house maintenance team. For some weeks, I was tasked with sawing white asbestos sheets into smaller squares for insertion into various piping ducts to upgrade the fire precautions. This was done in a small unventilated garage using a circular saw. I wore no mask. At the end of the day I was covered from head to foot in asbestos dust (the dangers of blue and brown asbestos were known but those of white asbestos had yet to be fully appreciated and legislation to protect workers did not come into being until the mid-1970's). Sometimes on the way home I would stop off, still in my working clothes, at the local pub for a drink which was tolerated if the taproom bar was used. Doubtless I contaminated that bar to what would now be considered dangerous levels!

University Hall was a standard traditional University Halls of Residence. If you arrived back late at night, the front door was locked and had to be opened upon request by the night Porter, ensconced in his lodge. This was not a problem but you had to sign in. Rumour had it that if you failed exams but had worked diligently, some sympathy would be given. However, if you failed exams and your name appeared too frequently on the late-entry register it would count against you. Similarly, you had to sign in for lectures. You obviously signed yourself in to the lectures with the right name but few people signed the late-entry register with their true names. Donald Duck and Mickey Mouse if scrawled in a drunken hand normally looked authentic. There were a number of wings in University Hall, with the slightly better accommodation being commandeered by those in their third year of the standard non-medical degree courses. The buildings were unisex, with the female students being accommodated in a tower block with en-suite wash basins. They had communal toilets and bathrooms down the corridor. The pathways below that tower block were littered with used condoms. Because of the access to a sink within the room, it had become common practice for the used condom to be filled with water, tied off and hurled out of windows onto unsuspecting passers-by. {Few single women were "on the pill" in 1971. Those who were could often be identified by the presence of chloasma. These were small patches of subtle increased pigmentation usually on the face and other areas exposed to sunlight which waxed and waned according to the season. The amount of oestrogen in the modern pills is now less and chloasma are now usually only seen during pregnancy. When I mentioned this little-known fact years later on a ward round, young medical students reckoned that some subcutaneous contraceptive implants would glow under disco lighting! Condoms were the mainstay of contraception at that time and had replaced the Coca-Cola douches of legend! An earlier generation of students had apparently relied upon the acidity therein being spermicidal with the classic glass bottle providing a convenient "shake and shoot" applicator.}

CHAPTER THREE

The Clinical Years

The two years spent at University Hall, preparing for the second MB, had been more of a standard type university-type education, with no patient contact and minimal exposure to actual medicine. This all changed in the autumn of 1973 and our ongoing education/training occurred mostly on the Heath campus where the medical school was based close to the hospital. There were also clinical attachments particularly to Llandough and Cardiff Royal Infirmary. The terms became longer, the holidays shorter and we started to feel like proper trainee doctors. I moved into the Hall of Residence above the Med Club bar and for the first time I had an en-suite basin; the bathrooms and toilets were down the corridor. We mostly ate out but there were reasonably well equipped kitchens on each floor. The Campus was vast and large numbers of trainees of various professions were living in. There were canteens and there was a nurse's home, in fact there were two or three situated in tower blocks, most of which were connected to the main hospital via service tunnels, such that you could walk about the site protected from the elements.

The Med Club bar was a lively place. There were formal discos, impromptu parties and a great deal of high-jinx often normally fuelled by alcohol. Behind the bar rested a three-pint pewter tankard. Periodically (and surprisingly frequently) there were challenges to see who could drain this tankard, which had been filled with cold lager, the fastest. For many, many years, the record was held by a medical student called Patrick, who, if I remember correctly, could do this in thirteen seconds. The usual method was for him to stand close to a plastic bin in the centre of the floor and drink whilst everybody hummed the 'Dam Busters March'. Three pints of cold gaseous liquid hitting a warm stomach had the predictable effect of causing almost instant vomiting hopefully aimed into the strategically placed bin (Vomiting – it is better to have an empty house, than an angry tenant).

These were part of the initiation ceremonies designed to make us feel one of the tribe. It was very early in the autumn of 1973 that I met my future wife Linda, who was a qualified nurse. She had recently moved to the Nurse's Home at the Heath, having trained in Swansea. She and her friend had drifted over to Med Club for a quiet drink. I was there with my own pals, doing nothing much in particular. Apparently, her friend fancied me but was too shy to make any approach. Their plan, apparently, was for Linda, who had more confidence, to make the initial approach. However, things got busy, the girls began to talk to others and I moved to sit some distance away. The first I heard was a voice calling out to alert me to the fact that I had dropped my pipe, which had rolled under a chair. That was Linda and that, as they say, was the start of it all. It however was almost thwarted. In the first few weeks of our relationship I took her to University Hall to meet up with my non-medic pals. Gwynfor was there and he and Linda recognised one another – they were second cousins. Apparently, he felt family loyalty transcended friendship and tried to put her off me by exaggerating my repute as the "mad medic" Fortunately he failed. I am reminded that the Seventeenth Century clergyman, Jeremy Taylor, described love as "friendship set on fire"; certainly as true now, as all those years ago.

Young doctors and nurses worked extremely long busy hours in those days and the general approach taken was to work hard and play hard. At some point, I read some nursing memoirs, which had an unfortunate spelling mistake. If I remember correctly, the quote went as follows: "When I was nursing in the 60's assisting the doctors and medical students was pure penile servitude".

Our clinical attachments involved a couple of days a week on the ward, with the rest of the time in lectures, the third year of which involved studying pathology and bacteriology. These were straightforward as academic subjects but I had a slight edge when it came to bacteriology. Linda had been heavily involved with a case of gas-gangrene on her ward and was using barrier nursing. I, of course had never heard of barrier nursing and Linda educated me. When an appropriate question came up in my examination, in addition to being able to deal and write about that which I ought to have known, I was able to add a short paragraph upon aspects of barrier nursing and infection control. That, I think, tipped the balance and got me a distinction in those two subjects.

As a clinical apprentice, there is a great deal to learn. Our guide was 'The Clinical Apprentice' by Naish, Read and Burns-Cox. This was basically a hand book of bedside manner, history taking and examination technique, which, in conjunction with bedside teaching from assorted doctors, mostly consultants, set us on the appropriate road. Charismatic bedside teachers included Paul Smith and Byron Evans. The neurologist John Graham was always smartly dressed and would demonstrate neurological examination on suitable patients at the weekly "Grand Round". We learned the very simple things initially, such as always approach the bed from the patient's right side and the basic principles of examination, which start with inspection, palpation, percussion and auscultation, which are generally applicable to every part of the body. There were a few alternative techniques, such as trans-illumination applied if there was doubt as to whether a mass in the scrotum was solid or cystic. If there was solid material in there, light would not pass through, whereas, if it was full of fluid, the light would pass through so called trans-illumination (I remember an Anaesthetist whispering in my ear in theatre, saying that the reason surgeons wore caps whilst operating was to stop the theatre lights trans-illuminating their empty skulls). I also recall an incident many years later, whilst I was examining some students on clinical technique. A female student had done a perfectly competent examination of a man's scrotum where there was a testicular swelling but completed the examination by listening to the scrotum with a stethoscope – not a recognised part of the examination of that area. I asked: "What did you hear?" To which she replied: "Normal scrotal sounds Sir" – there was frankly no answer to that. We were attached to clinical firms once we had been taught how to take bloods and sometimes assigned tasks to assist and ease the burden of the junior doctors.

In those days, staffing matters were much more formally structured. A typical ward of some thirty patients would have two consultants. Each consultant would have a middle grade registrar, a newly qualified pre-registration house officer and probably a senior house officer. If the consultants had particular skills to impart, there would often be a senior registrar shared between them. Senior house officers were up to two or three years qualified, registrars were anything between four and six years qualified and senior registrars could have been qualified some ten years and were awaiting consultant positions.

Standards were generally very high, particularly in surgery but, as in every walk of life, mistakes happened. The difference from then to now is that they were not always admitted with the candour that is required today. You will have heard of 'never events', those things that should never happen, such as removing the wrong limb or operating on the wrong side. There are system checks to prevent these, which are normally effective, though nothing can entirely eliminate human error. I remember going to theatre as a student, to watch a routine hernia repair. The patient was anaesthetised and on the table. Because the patient was lying on his back, the inguinal hernia had actually retracted under gravity and was not visible. The medical records were extremely sloppy and it was not crystal clear whether it was a right hernia or a left hernia. Mr Butcher, the Surgeon, made his incision in the right groin. Almost immediately, the Senior House officer (SHO) piped up, 'Sir, it's the other side'. 'No, it's not', said the Registrar. Well, I suppose we could have woken him up and asked him but the Anaesthetist had a better solution, he dripped some water down the endotracheal tube, making the patient cough. That revealed the hernia on the left side. 'Oh well' said Mr Butcher and extended his right incision across the abdomen, into the left. The hernia was duly repaired. On the post-op ward round, Mr Butcher shook the patient's hand and said 'I have done an excellent job on that one and while I was there, I inspected the other side as well and it's fine'. Those are the sort of actions, which today would have you struck off.

I also recall that there were serious problems with insulin intolerance in the early 70s. The only insulin available was beef insulin, prepared from the pancreas glands of slaughtered cattle. For most people, there was good tolerance but some people would develop antibodies, such that the dose of insulin necessary had to be increased and increased again, until heroic quantities were required. I recall a young man coming to the end of the road and told that there was no more that could be done. He chose to spend his last few weeks being as active as possible, with pleasures centred upon women and beer.

Around that time, the Professor of bacteriology, Professor Scott-Thompson, retired. There was a 'do' put on for him at lunchtime, with some food. Although I did not know him well, I tagged along and learned a fascinating fact, as follows: Wartime Prime Minister, Winston Churchill, had been taken ill in North Africa, with pneumonia. The then Major Scott-Thompson RAMC was dispatched on the dangerous journey, courtesy of the RAF, with apparently half the world's supply of penicillin in his briefcase. Churchill's treating physicians were reluctant to use an experimental drug and continued with the Sulphonamides and Churchill survived. As I recall the tale, that penicillin was considered too valuable to risk losing on the return journey, should disaster befall and was put to good use in a British field hospital, mostly treating German prisoners of war, with apparently great success. {As an aside, Alexander Fleming, by accident, identified that penicillin was an effective antibiotic back in 1928. There was, however a problem in producing it because it grew so slowly. Apparently, a major breakthrough happened again by accident in 1943, when a laboratory worker in Illinois brought in some mouldy cantaloupe melons from the local market. They were infected with a type of penicillium which yielded about twice as much penicillin as Fleming's original strain. Another bacteriologist in Wisconsin, Dr McCoy, discovered that by irradiating this mould, she could produce a mutant strain, which was a thousand times more productive and paved the way for the commercial production of all subsequent penicillins. Because penicillin was in such short supply, it was normally recovered from the urine of patients, for reuse later. For obvious reasons, it was being used for military purposes, particularly for gunshot and shrapnel wounds. Many soldiers convalescing in field hospitals were allowed beer as a 'medicinal comfort'. Unfortunately, this increased the volume of urine and made the process of recovering the penicillin more complex. These troops were therefore banned from drinking beer and this led to the belief that alcohol should not be consumed with antibiotics}. Shrapnel nowadays refers to random bits of metal embedded in the body following explosions. It is not a German word. A young British Royal Artillery officer in the 19th Century, Henry Shrapnel, invented a spherical case (shrapnel shells) containing musket balls mixed with explosive. These would explode scattering the balls widely. For the wife, shrapnel in the wrong place could seriously wreck her plans!

The essential key to making a diagnosis is firstly obtained from elucidating a good history. The actual facts need to be established in a fairly logical and structured manner. Firstly, you ask about the presenting complaint and set that against the background of previous medical history and medication being taken. You then do a brief system enquiry by asking questions related to the cardiovascular system, the central nervous system, the gastro-enterological system and the urological system. This ought to pick up incidentals and helps direct the subsequent physical examination. When all the facts have been gathered, the astute doctor, using the hard-learned knowledge of pathology, crafted a differential diagnosis. This formed the basis of further testing to exclude rarities and hopefully confirm a final diagnosis. So, it's history, examination and then tests. A useful way of looking at this is by comparing it to betting on a horse. The test on its own is merely the stable-boy's tip, which, on its own, may or may not be relevant or accurate. The racing equivalent to the history is studying the form from previous performance, with the equivalent of examination being actually watching the horse perform in the field. Diagnostic accuracy is enhanced if all three are done thoroughly. Over recent years there has been an increasing trend to reverse this by doing a battery of tests first and then focussing history taking and examination around the abnormalities identified.

My pal Stan and I were charged with taking a student history from a lady who was in hospital, awaiting removal of a gallbladder. {Gallstones were said to predominate in those who were Fair, Fat, Female, Forty and Fertile} She undoubtedly had gallstones but her history of recurrent nausea, (without much pain) and recurrent vomiting, was somewhat atypical. We discovered that she had a very low pulse rate at 50 beats per minute and her blood pressure was persistently high. She also complained of headaches. Now, we knew very little being junior medical students but the combination of nausea, high blood pressure and reduced pulse, especially if associated with headaches, is suggestive of raised intracranial pressure, perhaps due to a brain tumour. When we presented this case to the consultant at a teaching ward round; there was a bit of jaw dropping, followed by a more detailed examination of the back of the retina with an ophthalmoscope and indeed, there were signs highly suggestive of raised intracranial pressure. This set in train a cancelled unnecessary cholecystectomy and the diagnosis of a brain tumour. Back in the 70s there were no CT or MRI scans and even ultrasound scans were unavailable in most hospitals before 1975. By the standards of today, the diagnostic tools were primitive. There were isotope scans and clever neurological x-rays, such as air encephalograms, which were exceptionally painful for the patient and whilst they gave good results by the standard of the time, they were superseded and became obsolete.

The Medical Hall of Residence above the Med Club was a tower block, I think nine stories high. A favourite ploy when bored was to fill black bin bags with water (they were stronger in those days than now) – tie them off and hurl them out of the windows. Normally, they would land with a reassuring bang on the roof of Med Club, which was a ground floor extension slightly to one side. Just occasionally, they would miss and land on the ground, soaking anyone within about twelve feet; we could normally get three gallons into a bin bag. No one was injured but on one occasion, a rather battered student mini had its roof caved in.

Med Club fulfilled all the fire regulations and had conveniently placed fire hoses. Although not done often, high jinks would occasionally require that those fire hoses were put to use in water fights. Unbeknown to us initially, the unreeling of a fire hose triggered a fire alarm and being a hospital site, prompted the arrival of numerous fire engines. Whether or not the hospital had to pay for fire engine attendance, as they do now, is uncertain but the practice was absolutely banned after someone turned the firehose on the approaching firemen. We were reminded that as clinical medical students, we were effectively on some form of General Medical Council pre-register and sanctions could be applied upon qualification. My pal Stan had a criminal record for petty larceny, having pinched a geranium plant from a display in the foyer of a Cardiff hotel, where some examination successes were being celebrated. In effect, the hotel had laid out a beautiful display of geraniums in pots and as students left, they each picked one up, such that the absence of geraniums was total by one o'clock in the morning. The manager called the police and whilst the police probably didn't take it seriously, they spotted Stan acting suspiciously, sitting on a wall by a bus stop – the buses had long since ceased for the night. When they asked him what he was doing and asked him to move on, he stooped down, picked up the geranium and started to stagger on his way. That was a 'red rag to a bull' and he was nicked. I also recall interviewing for a consultant post many years later. The candidate was absolutely excellent and ideally suited to the job. The panel had asked all the relevant questions and I, as 'tail end Charlie' had really nothing of any use to ask. As I idly

63

flicked through his application form, I noticed that the section on 'Criminal Record' had actually been completed (for certain jobs, particularly medicine and nursing, convictions are never spent). I asked him to outline his past, as a master criminal. There was a look of shock around the table, until he confessed that he had a criminal record for riding a bicycle without lights, dating from his student days. When asked why he had bothered to put it down, he gave his reason. Had he not declared it, he would have technically lied on the application form and could have been dismissed at the whim of his employer. He considered it more prudent to confess upfront. A very wise move!

As the course progressed formal lectures decreased and we spent increasing time on the wards, acquiring the essential clinical skills. Anyone late for a teaching ward round would be likened to "an undescended testicle" – late in arriving, problematic and useless upon arrival. Whilst dress-code was not over strictly enforced, we were expected to dress like young professionals and men were expected to wear ties on clinical attachment (in contrast to today, when ties have been banned, along with white coats and long sleeved shirts). The first two years with no clinical contact had been much more relaxed, though most people were relatively tidy. The 'hippy era' had passed but, mainly in other faculties, there were some extremely hippy-like characters. This reminds me of a comment by Ronald Reagan on hippies: "Look like Tarzan, walk like Jane, smell like Cheetah".

As we gained clinical skills, it was common practice for the more diligent to hang around the casualty department (now known as A&E), at Cardiff Royal Infirmary, in the hope of seeing some interesting conditions. If you were prepared to hang around late at night, or over the weekend, you often got to assist junior surgeons in theatre and acquire some extra-curricular teaching. I recall a young man being admitted with what turned out to be an abscess around a recently removed appendix. His appendix had been removed for acute appendicitis some two weeks earlier, whilst he was abroad on holiday and he had returned to the UK, seemingly well. On the basis of a fever, a high white cell count and extreme tenderness over the appendix scar, he went immediately to theatre for an exploratory operation. There was indeed a large abscess, the centre of which was a gauze swab, left behind during his previous operation. I am not sure if the surgeon realised that his original operation had been abroad but nonetheless, he called for a new set of gloves and deftly and by sleight of hand lost the swab into the folded down old glove, which was discarded into the bin and as such did not feature as an extra in the swab count. The abscess was cleaned up, antibiotics prescribed and the patient made an uneventful recovery. When I asked the surgeon afterwards what he was playing at, he indicated that it was probably better to lose the swab, rather than cause the team who had left it in any medico-legal difficulties. Again, the probability is that one would be struck off nowadays for such activities. Life in Med Club continued to be enjoyable. Various girlfriends became almost fixtures and one of the younger ward sisters would often turn up in uniform at the end of her shift, around 9 pm; her specialty, after a few drinks, was to strip off whilst dancing on the piano, much to the amusement of all. On particularly high-spirited nights, many people did this and it was generally known as a "Zumba", done to a chorus of singing.

Rugby was a popular game in both the medical school and South Wales in general. The medical school first team was certainly up to standard in playing local clubs and indeed, some Welsh international players were actually part of the faculty and team. Whenever rugby internationals were played, the television was moved to pride of place in the bar, seats gathered round and the festivities commenced. International matches in Scotland particularly but also Dublin would be visited, if tickets could be obtained. The procedure for the Edinburgh trip had been well rehearsed and the spectators usually headed off, some four or five days before the match. Medical student contacts in Birmingham, Liverpool and Manchester would provide en-route accommodation on their floors in reciprocity for similar accommodation for internationals played in Cardiff. Occasionally, friendly rugby matches were played, though more usually matters degenerated into a beer fest. The essential ingredients for a successful trip were the hiring of a coach and the capture of a milk churn from outside a farmer's entrance gate. The churn provided a suitably capacious receptacle for urine and vomit along the way and could be conveniently emptied periodically down a grid. Beer barrels and glasses were loaded onto the coach and operated by foot pumps. A law student, who had tagged along, always maintained that it was perfectly legal to urinate off the rear off-side wheel of a coach when stationary on the street. Whether this was the case and whether the law has been repealed, I know not but popular wisdom suggested that it was only applicable if the town in question had been a recognised coaching town from the days of stage coaches. It was on one such trip like this that a ten pound bet was made. The circumstances were as follows: the individual concerned was an excellent and diligent student. By facial appearance, he looked a little strange at first sight and potentially looked a little mad. His party piece was to act 'Schizophrenic'. He was very good at it. The bet was that for ten pounds, he could get himself sectioned under the old Mental Health Act. At some point on the trip, he presented himself to a casualty department, outside Liverpool. It may have been Whiston Hospital; it may have been Broadgreen Hospital. He paced around the waiting room, talking what he deemed 'schizophrenic', which attracted the attention of the staff. In due course, phone calls were made and white coated attendants bundled him into an ambulance. The upshot was that he was indeed sectioned and taken to the large psychiatric hospital at Rainhill. The rugby trip moved on, went to Edinburgh, came back and normality was restored, except, our friend was absent without leave. No one knew where he actually was. When you were attached to wards and expected to do clinical duties, absence was noticed. Matters were covered up for a couple of days with lame excuses. Now, some of our teachers were relatively junior doctors, who we had known from their student days. They were reasonably approachable. We approached a young registrar and explained that our chappie was perhaps still in Rainhill Hospital under a Section Order. He phoned one of his friends, who was a junior psychiatrist and the seriousness of the situation soon became apparent. We were paraded in front of the Professor and Dean of the medical school, where the facts were relayed, as best as possible. "So boys, you think he's got himself sectioned into Rainhill Hospital and is still there"? "Yes" we replied. There was a lot of tut, tut, tutting and we were dismissed. Apparently, the Dean then phoned Rainhill Hospital, got hold of the psychiatrist responsible and explained that there had been a prank. The psychiatrist's version of the story was that our friend had been put in a padded cell on admission and had dozed off. The following morning, he had bragged to a charge nurse that he was actually a medical student from Cardiff, getting himself sectioned for a bet. The charge nurse, apparently a wily fellow, had heard it all before, so our friend was duly heavily sedated. That was still the situation which pertained at the time of the phone call. The psychiatrist maintained that this was a legal order, made with good reason and that he would have to serve his full twenty-eight day section-term for observation. This was duly done. He finally returned back a month later to much clapping and the sight of yellow ribbons tied around the bushes. Some prissy people, including my future wife, thought that this was an appalling waste of NHS resources but the rest of us thought it was highly amusing. However, there was a sting in the tale.

It soon became apparent that the Section Order along with reasons for it, had been communicated to his General Practitioner and formed an integral part of his medical record. So, when, in due course, he applied for a mortgage and appropriate life assurance, this was denied on the basis that he was potentially at significant risk of either suicide, risky behaviour or general defaulting upon debts. Whether this was ever fully sorted out, I know not but that was still the situation some twelve or more years after the incident. He did, however, win his ten pounds. At some point on campus, the mother of Wayne Scales, who was a midwife, attended a refresher course on the Heath Campus. She was provided with accommodation on the third or fourth floor of the nurses' home. Her husband, a fiery retired military officer came to visit. The porter on the lodge of the nurses' home would not let him in but not to be thwarted, he obtained a rope from the back of the car, arranged for it to be smuggled up to his wife and climbed up and gained entry.

In addition to ward work, we were attached to general practitioners. They had obviously been carefully selected and gave us a somewhat rose-tinted view of general practice. I was attached to a practice of two middle aged, extremely genteel and competent GPs in one of the more affluent suburbs of Cardiff. Life then was much more relaxed. There was no appointment system and patients turned up and were seen. It seemed more art than science. I recall one mother concerned about her son's vague leg pains being told that it was nothing serious – just his undescended toes which were still trying to wriggle out to their full extent. Similarly perceived bandy-legs were treated by wearing the shoes on the wrong feet. They must have read Voltaire, "The art of medicine is to amuse the patient whilst the disease cures itself". At least no harm was done or unnecessary investigations performed for these self-limiting conditions. Surgery started at about nine o'clock; there was half hour break at half past ten, when tea and biscuits were served and surgery normally finished before midday. The handful of home visits was done on the way home to a sumptuous roast dinner, prepared by their wives. The afternoon was spent reading the paper or mostly dozing on the settee, awaiting the start of evening surgery at about five o'clock. All was finished at half past seven and then we were homeward bound. The Professor of General Practice had a model practice, centred upon a council estate on the periphery of Cardiff. He worked as a general practitioner and was well supported by senior academics in general practice. He drove a very large car, a Bentley I think. Everything in that practice ran impeccably to order, with no stresses. The patients were well behaved, doctors not overstretched and it was a particularly idyllic attachment. However, one of our number, Evan, complained bitterly that he wished to see 'real' general practice, as he was used to back home in the somewhat impoverished Welsh Valley communities. The Professor was somewhat taken aback by this request, as all the general practitioners to whom we were attached had been carefully selected to give the best possible impression. However, true to his word, he phoned around and contacted Evan, informing him that he had arranged for him to be attached for a short period to a general practitioner in the Rhondda. Evan arrived on the train, to be met at the station by his new tutor riding a bicycle, with a spare one for Evan. It turned out that his tutor was an alcoholic who had lost his driving licence. All home visits were done on a bicycle. Whilst no one doubted the medical competency of the doctor, his social life was in disarray. Evan was further surprised to find that a satellite surgery was regularly held in a small village in the public bar of the local hostelry. Evan already had a dim view of general practice and this experience just exacerbated matters and the first thing he did upon qualification was join the Canadian Military and move abroad.

Although we spent relatively little time in any laboratories, we occasionally did some bacteriology. This would often involve plating up some pus on a petri dish and seeing if we could incubate and identify the bacteria. At one such practical, we had been provided with a range of pus from various sources and appropriate swabs. We worked in pairs, all quiet and straightforward. Suddenly, consternation and fisticuffs broke out in the lab. It turned out that when one pair of male students were swabbing the throats of each other to plate out, one had used, instead of a nice fresh clean swab, one that had already been soaking in gonorrhoea pus. I would imagine that it was all sorted out with antibiotics but I am glad that incident did not happen to me. Central to the Heath Hospital was a large concourse, with shops, seating areas, coffee bars and facilities, such as a bank branch. It was a very convivial and convenient place to meet up and while away the odd spare hour, whilst still being on site. One lunch time, a young doctor moved a table to the centre and stood upon it and began auctioning his possessions for charity. Bids were trivial but nonetheless, he sold his car, he sold his television, he sold his radio, he then went to sell his stethoscope, his white coat, his tie, his shirt, his shoes and his socks. By the time he was half-naked someone got hold of one of his friends; the upshot of which was that he had had a psychiatric breakdown due to bipolar disorder. He was admitted as a voluntary patient to psychiatry and underwent quite extensive treatment.

One of our attachments on a modular basis was for occupational health. This is a very important part of medicine and has contributed to a great deal of health and safety in the work place. A few trips were arranged to liven things up. A bunch of males (females aren't allowed down pits), visited a local mine. We descended in the cage to be met by large tunnels, big enough to drive small trucks around. The coal seam was a long way from the pit head. As the tunnels narrowed we noticed that loose planks covered in white dust were periodically balanced across the passages. Apparently, these were designed such that if there was an explosion underground, the dust would immediately be shaken off and minimise the risk of any fire spreading. Mining was a very dangerous activity. Coal dust was everywhere and many miners developed crippling emphysema from pneumoconiosis – although masks were available few used them as they impaired breathing. Gases of various types dangerously seeped into mines and were known as the "Damps". Black damp – lack of oxygen; white damp – carbon monoxide; fire damp – methane and stink damp – hydrogen sulphide. This latter gas, typically used in stink-bomb pranks at school or church, was potentially lethal when it reached high concentrations. The rule of thumb was that if you could smell the odour of "rotten eggs" concentrations were relatively low, whereas the ability to detect it by smell was lost at high concentration. Most miners acquired coal dust "tattooing" from dust getting into cuts and scratches.

As the course advanced and relationships firmed up, there were a number of marriages in our year. Linda and I got married some six months before I qualified, simply because it was more convenient to do it then, rather than try to do everything, including start working, within a few weeks of actually qualifying. We managed to avoid some of the classic excesses of stag nights but I do recall someone who acquired a plaster of Paris cast on their stag night (for no good reason, other than a prank) and was actually allowed to go up the aisle wearing it. They did of course have the decency to take it off before he went on honeymoon. His wife was not amused.

CHAPTER FOUR

The Junior Doctor Years

Theodore Roosevelt is quoted as saying "The best prize that life has to offer is the chance to work hard at work worth doing". An antique mirror restorer once mused that his was a job he could always see himself doing! Anyway, come July 1976, I had qualified and embarking on the next adventure. This was akin to passing the driving test. The examiner has deemed that you are competent about the basics but you know deep down that there is still a lot to learn. Our clinical course had been mostly modular, with exams of some description virtually every six weeks. Therefore, as a result, the actual final examinations were not as daunting as they had been to previous generations. Our knowledge was, however tested in written format and by the presentation of history, clinical signs and differential diagnoses, following the clinical examination of patients. Some were on the wards being treated but many had volunteered to come in especially in order to show off their signs and symptoms. Most of us had voluntarily prepared for qualification by doing 'student locums'. In effect, you took over the role of one of the junior house officers, who was on holiday, and muddled on as best you could. The ward sister would normally give tactful advice or resist complying with dangerous activities/suggestions. Other junior doctors were always available to provide help.

I did my six month medicine at Llandough Hospital on the "firm" of Paul Smith, general physician/gastro-enterologist, who had some 15 patients spread between two unisex wards. House officers paired up and we worked a one-in-two rota. We both worked the standard forty-hour week, thereafter one of us had to be available on-site to cover the remaining hundred and twenty-eight hours of the week. Typically, on your 'heavy' week, you only had thirty-two hours off out of the whole week. Typically, this would be the hours between 5.00 pm on a Tuesday and 9.00 am on a Wednesday and 5.00 pm on a Thursday to 09.00 am on a Friday. The rest of the time you were resident on-call. On your 'lighter' week you were only on call for those thirty-two hours, but there was no routine holiday cover so if one was on leave and no student locum could be secured you were tied to the hospital 24/7 for the duration. By the standards of today, we were not necessarily busy after midnight and not every one of those nights on-call was involved in seeing new emergency patients. Other wards were also being covered by their resident house officers. The living accommodation in the mess at Llandough was old fashioned but very comfortable. A cup of tea was normally brought to your door at about 08.00 in the morning and there were pleasant facilities to relax within, if things were slack. On the odd occasional when you were also on-call for new patients, as well as covering your wards, it could be extremely busy, but most nights you could be assured of three to four hours uninterrupted sleep.

There had been a junior doctors' strike in 1975, which had ensured that on-call time was subsequently paid. Because it was deemed on-call and not really work, the hourly rate was paid at 30% of the standard hourly rate. {When doctors strike all the scientific evidence suggests that patients stop dying (Cunningham S A, Mitchell K et al. Doctor' strikes and mortality: a review. Soc Sci Med 2008; 67:1784-1788). It seems that the key reason is that elective surgery ceases and it is this non-emergency work which carries a surprisingly high mortality rate. A possible conclusion is that the public and probably also doctors themselves overestimate the ability of medicine to influence mortality. Alternatively, and because even during strikes some emergency care is always provided, it may be that when doctors refuse to follow orders and conform to employer's restrictive practises, they practise a freer type of medicine which is better for patients!}

Because we were constantly available on-site, we were exposed to a great deal and climbed a very steep learning curve. Mistakes attracted humiliating public bollockings, often on ward rounds, designed to teach us the errors of our ways. Colourful tirades of verbal abuse doubtless taught us resilience. One ex-army surgeon once let fly with a wonderful set of threats involving castration with a blunt knife, then partial garrotting to be followed by firing squad if that mistake ever happened again! It turned out that he had received the same bollocking as a junior officer in Normandy in 1944 and had committed it to memory. It is said that good judgement comes from experience and experience comes from having made the errors of judgement yourself.

Often, we lacked the experience to know whether or not, if complications arose, we had caused them, or whether these problems were inevitable.

One middle aged man was admitted with a pneumothorax. A tear had spontaneously developed at the periphery of his lung, such that air escaped from the lung with each breath, entering the chest cavity. The upshot was that with each breath, more air entered the chest and resulted in the lung progressively collapsing. He was short of breath, the percussion note on that side was hyper resonant (more drum-like than the other) and the diagnosis was confirmed by chest x-ray. The standard procedure was to insert a tube into the chest wall. This would let out the air and if attached to an underwater seal drain, prevent the air from returning. With luck, the lung would re-expand and the hole in it spontaneously repair. In fact, all went well, apart from the recognised complication of subcutaneous emphysema. Where the tube entered the chest, air began to seep under the skin. It tracked everywhere and within a few hours, he was blown up like the 'Michelin man'. I thought that I had done something wrong only to discover from the 'wise' that this was a non-harmful complication, which would resolve in time. It duly did, as the air was reabsorbed. I learned that professional guilt is in effect letting someone live in your head rent free!

A young student was admitted with jaundice under another team. He had suffered from a flu-like illness over the previous few days and had turned yellow. Hepatitis was suspected but excluded. He was not systemically unwell and had no temperature but remained jaundiced. There was no bile detected in his urine. Someone suspected gallstones (very unusual in a young male) and organised the standard test of the day, an oral cholecystogram. In simple terms, if you had a gallbladder full of stones, then the stones would prevent the gallbladder filling up with the dye taken orally as part of the test. When x-rayed, the gallbladder would appear non-functional and by inference suggest the presence of stones. The test was duly done and no dye appeared in the gallbladder. He had been placed on the list for a cholecystectomy by his surgeon. I vaguely knew this student and was having a brief chat with him when Paul Smith came over. We happened to discuss the case very briefly and Paul made the correct diagnosis. In fact, this young man did not have gallstones; he had a rather common condition, known as Gilbert's syndrome. {Some 5% of the population have it and it is normally inconsequential} These individuals have a problem metabolising the bilirubin that enters bile, such that they always have a slightly high blood level of bilirubin but too low to manifest itself as actual jaundice visible to the eye. Any general malaise or flu-like illness can disrupt matters and produce the classic yellow appearance of jaundice. It is also the pathway for the dye taken for an oral cholecystogram. Basically, the wrong diagnosis was made initially simply because he had this metabolic defect.

In general, we were closely supervised and subtly guided by the experienced ward sisters. Common things occurred commonly and fairly quickly, we became confident in dealing with the routine conditions. We had been warned very early as students that much of what we would be taught would be proven to be wrong and even that which was not wrong, would be made obsolete by advances in medical knowledge. All this indeed came to pass. Surgical house jobs followed at Cardiff Royal

Infirmary and at the Heath, with a two month period spent as a junior ENT surgeon. My role was primarily limited to the removal of foreign bodies which had found themselves up the noses and into the ears of young children. Tonsillectomies were still popular treatments, normally swiftly done using a specific guillotine, rather than dissection. Over the course of the day, a bin full of tonsils would be acquired. Apparently, they made useful fishing bait and were often taken home by keen anglers. One young man with a stocky neck did not thrive too well after his tonsillectomy. He became weaker and more lethargic. There seemed to be no obvious cause for this but when I checked his blood count, his haemoglobin had dropped to five grams (a third of what it was on admission). I had failed to recognise that he had been bleeding slowly from the tonsillectomy wound and required a transfusion.

We learnt the lessons of what they do not teach in medical school. I share some of them as follows:

- A quick test for dehydration or a reduced albumin level was to inject saline subcutaneously, sufficient to raise a bump of fluid. In the presence of dehydration this would be rapidly absorbed and vanish. If the albumin level was low, there would be lack of osmotic pressure and the raised lump would persist.

- If postoperative patients were leaking fluid from their wound, a quick test to see whether this was from an abnormal connection with the gut (fistula) or merely infection, was to dip a piece of blackened x-ray film in the discharge. If it was a fistula (containing proteinases) the x-ray film would whiten as the blackened silver fell off when the protein on the film dissolved.

- It is always wise to give a guarded prognosis, regardless of the condition. By so doing, you prepare the road for complications, whereas a flamboyant "Ah, he'll be fine" can give the impression of being uncaring and cavalier.

- There is no such thing as minor surgery – only minor surgeons.

- Experienced doctors know what they don't know. In essence, they are wise enough to know their own limitations.

- Hospitals are intrinsically bad places, especially for the elderly. A wrong differential diagnosis can lead to tests, the results of which can expand, rather than reduce the differential diagnosis and beget more and more investigations. Essentially, they become the victims of medical investigation technology, known as "VOMIT". Iatrogenic illness and drug errors can add to detriment. Patients can fall; they may be assaulted by other patients and catch infections. Mild confusion due to illness can worsen in the noisy alien environment of a ward, exacerbated by loss of hearing aids, glasses and false teeth. This can accelerate the spiral of decline, leading to an erroneous diagnosis of dementia (detain me if you please!). This in turn precludes the return home and precipitation of long-term care.

- All medications have side effects. If those side effects require further drugs to relieve symptoms, this can lead to a spiral of over-prescription.

- Whether somebody is fit to discharge can be determined by the 'fire alarm test'. Simply, set off the fire alarm, those who can reach the door in a timely manner are fit for discharge.

- To differentiate the common cold from flu, put a £10 note on the floor. Those who can get up and retrieve it do not have flu.

- The dose of any medication is one or two tablets or five or ten mls of fluid. If the dose you have calculated turns out to be significantly higher than that, it is wrong until proven otherwise.

- We will all make mistakes. It is not the mistake that will get you into trouble, it is the cover-up.

- Today's miracle cure may turn out to be tomorrow's poison.

- The good that doctors do in their careers will turn out to be much less than they thought that they would do.

- Screening can cause more problems than it will solve. If it aint broke, don't fix it.

- Always treat the patient, not the test result.

- Old age is associated with wisdom. Sadly, it can be unaccompanied.

- A sick baby is a sick baby when the mother says it is.

- Demented drivers who lack insight into their conditions can be an absolute menace on the roads. If on a domiciliary visit you need to disable a car, the "quick fix" is to ram a potato onto the exhaust pipe. This either prevents the engine starting or causes it to cut out fairly smartly. If you can get inside the bonnet, you can remove the distributor cap or the king lead.

- In the absence of an underwater seal drain, a one-way non-return valve, akin to the Heimlich valve, can be improvised by tying a condom or the finger cut from a rubber glove, over the end of the tube, with the end cut off. As air is blown out, it goes out without impediment but as soon as air tries to return, the rubber tube will usually scrunch up and prevent air re-entry.

- The biggest risk factor for cancer is age; everything else is trivial in comparison.

- If you consult text books in front of patients, it will give the wrong impression. They will rarely think you are diligent, just ignorant.

- A doctor who lacks some diagnostic doubt can turn out to be an executioner.

- Individual doctors generate much of their workload.

- Never treat animals. Not only is it illegal as they lack the capacity to consent to irregular practitioners but some animals react to medications in different ways. I'm told that morphine stimulates cats and horses rather than sedates them. Vets however can treat people if the "patient" consents, knowing that they are vets.

- Above all, the practice of medicine should be fun.

The standard of medical school qualification in the UK is overseen by the General Medical Council (GMC).

The standard university qualification is with the degrees Bachelor of Medicine and Bachelor of Surgery. There is, however, an alternative qualification, the so-called conjoint diploma, granting the current qualification of LRCP and LRCS (Licentiate of the Royal Colleges of Physician/Surgeons). If I remember correctly, it was possible to sit the conjoint diploma some months prior to sitting the degree, in June. A handful of people tried to hedge their bets and protect against potential failure of the degree by sitting the conjoint and ensuring that qualification and the ability to do the pre-registration year was assured. Historically, the Worshipful Societies of Apothecaries of London and Dublin could issue their own primary medical qualifications, the LSA (Licentiate of the Society of Apothecaries). I believe the GMC declined to accept the Dublin LSA as a registerable qualification back in the early 70s but the LSA from London was acceptable for some years after I qualified. I knew of no one that had taken that qualification but some older doctors had the LSA as their sole qualification. Upon qualification, provisional registration with the GMC was granted. With a successful 12 months as pre-registration house officer behind one, you became fully registered.

The old General Medical Council was controlled predominately by doctors, with some lay members. It was interested in preserving the reputation of the profession. The actions which could bring trouble upon a registered doctor mostly began with 'A'. They included adultery with patients, abortion, addiction to drugs, alcoholism, advertising and association with Quacks (as an aside, the Dutch import 'quack' popped up in the vocabulary in the early 1700's to describe a medical charlatan. It was short for 'quacksalver', meaning

82

somebody who quacked their salves or cures. It had nothing to do with the beaked masks of the plague doctors (those masks were surprisingly effective in preventing the spread of airborne infection from coughs and sneezes). The modern GMC regulations are more patient-focused and have been progressively so since the GMC has acquired predominately lay membership. The focus on being a good doctor is centred upon competence, caring in the sense of taking care to avoid errors, communication, confidentiality, concordance in the sense of agreeing a plan with the patient and candour when things go wrong.

After a successful house officer year behind one, the next step was planning a future career. In my day, it was possible to move straight from house officer jobs into general practice, as a partner. Few did, the exceptions being those who could move into practice with a medical relative. Most aspiring general practitioners chose to do a couple of years in hospital, learning essential skills in paediatrics and obstetrics, together with medicine, before moving into general practice for a year's formal training in that specialty. Aspiring physicians and surgeons competed hotly for senior house officer posts in centres of excellence. Jobs were normally of six months duration, with no security of tenure. The result was that no sooner had you started one six month job, you were frantically looking for the next. This was extremely disruptive to anyone married. For those who were single and unattached, it was not particularly problematic; because of the frequency of on-call, accommodation was provided onsite and free. For those who were renting marital flats offsite and eager to get on the housing ladder, it was more difficult. There is no doubt that the teaching hospital posts would provide good training.

However, they were not necessarily sufficiently busy to provide a huge amount of experience. After much deliberation, I elected to train as a physician. In order to acquire some security of tenure, I applied for a two year rotational post in the North East of England. Although this was in district general hospitals, the medical standards were high and the training generally excellent. In the mid-70s inflation was roaring away and we took the plunge and bought a house. We were only in it some fifteen months before selling up and moving on, though we made 20% profit in that short period, providing a deposit for further properties as we ascended the property ladder. The move out of the teaching centres was a huge gamble, as it depended upon my acquiring the membership of the Royal College of Physicians, by examination. This was a costly examination to take and consisted of two parts, both of which had a high failure rate. It was not easy to find the time to study, working a one-in-three on-call rota, which was resident and having a new born baby to contend with at home. However, needs must and I was lucky to pass both parts of the examination at first attempt. By November 1978, I was a member of the Royal College of Physicians (UK) and still had some eight months to run on my contract. I was also able to apply for jobs if they came up at unusual times of the year. Most people moved jobs on the 1st August and the 1st February. Linda and I decided not to return to South Wales and we could not really afford to move to London. We were therefore limited to a handful of English teaching hospitals, as and when jobs were advertised. An ideal registrar post was advertised in Liverpool. I had suitable references, the full membership examination and was appointed as the registrar to the professorial unit, based at Broadgreen Hospital.

My gamble had paid off and although I only spent some twenty months in the North East, I gained a huge amount of experience, as they were far busier jobs than their equivalents would have been in the rarified atmosphere of the teaching hospital. Although not directly involved, there was the incident of a young man, coincidentally an amateur boxer, who was knifed in a street brawl. There were two tiny chest punctures, producing a tension pneumothorax on the right, which was appropriately diagnosed and treated with the insertion of a chest drain. He made no improvement and his blood pressure continued to fall. No one knew how long the blade with which he had been stabbed was but an abdominal bleed was suspected. Treatment then progressed to an abdominal laparotomy, with the standard incision from pubis to chest being made. No pathology was discovered. The incision was extended to his right arm pit and his chest opened. The pericardial sac, which surrounds the heart, was full of blood. This was opened, a small nick in the heart itself was repaired and the patient survived. Many months later, his picture appeared in the local newspaper. He was dressed in boxing shorts and adopting a pugilistic posture, which revealed the massive scar extending from his pubis to his right armpit. The headline read "Man survives stabbing in street brawl" giving the impression of a sabre attack.

Each day one of the local evening papers used to publish the names of hospital patients who were deemed to be critically ill. Anyone who survived would often carry on their person a dog-eared copy of the paper cutting as a" badge of office", being proud to announce 'I was on the list, doctor'.

Serious misdiagnoses occasionally occurred. On one occasion, a man in his fifties was admitted routinely for some procedure. He had been a diabetic for thirty years, on insulin and had led a quiet life. He had avoided stress and although bright, had never sought promotion in work. He had a very steady routine and his diabetes was impeccably well controlled. Whilst in hospital and for reasons I can't recall, his insulin was omitted for some two days. Surprisingly, his blood sugar level was quite normal, there were no ketones in his urine and he felt well. Spontaneous cure of diabetes after that period of time is almost unheard of. Further tests were done, which established beyond any doubt that he was not currently a diabetic. His old records were sought and obtained. Looking back, the diagnosis of diabetes, some thirty years before, had been made on exceptionally shaky grounds. His insulin was stopped and he was discharged without further problem. In retrospect, this man had been severely detrimented; for the previous thirty years; he had avoided sport, he had led a quiet life and he had never applied for a promotion, all because of a completely wrong diagnosis.

The classic symptoms of Parkinson's disease consist of the triad of a pill rolling tremor, muscle rigidity of the limbs and slowness in getting moving. The tremor is sometimes the most obvious sign but the least reliable when it comes to making the diagnosis. Treatment with medications, such as Sinemet and Madopar benefits the slowness of movement and muscular rigidity but often does little for the tremor.

As a general rule of thumb, Parkinson's disease is relentlessly progressive; leaving most suffers functionally very dependent within ten years of diagnosis. On many occasions, I have seen Parkinson's disease misdiagnosed when the symptoms and signs have really fitted best with a diagnosis of benign essential tremor. The tablets given have had no significant side effects but have done no particular good. Because the diagnosis was wrong, these individuals have not worsened over many, many years. On two occasions, I have seen articulate individuals, who, following the diagnosis, had joined the local Parkinson's Society for support. Two people had become the local chairmen of their Parkinson's Society and had held those positions for many years. One of them had done a great deal of good for the local Parkinson's Society and there was a moral dilemma as to whether he could rightfully continue to hold that position, if the diagnosis of Parkinson's disease was ultimately trashed. There was much debate as to whether it would be for the greater good to leave matters as they were or to reveal all.

Whilst in the North East, I was attached to a gastroenterologist, for some six months, as part of the rotation. One of the then tests for malabsorption was the so called three day faecal fat test. In essence, the patient collected three days' worth of faeces at home, in plastic containers, which then went to the laboratory to determine whether there was excess fat, suggesting poor absorption. One lady from an affluent suburb had duly collected three days' worth of faeces in three significantly large plastic tubs, which she had placed in a smart tartan bag. She elected to visit the hospital by public transport and when she put her bag on the floor whilst making some purchase in a shop, somebody nicked her bag. When she appeared in clinic and related this tale, we had great difficulty in keeping the smiles from our faces.

As a small child growing up in Stockport, I used to be fascinated watching steeple jacks, high up on factory chimneys; like tiny flies. The North East of England had similar extremely tall factory chimneys. Whilst doing a general medical clinic, a man attended, complaining of faints. He was also periodically a little weak, with occasional light-headedness. I gave him a thorough clinical examination, discovering a harsh cardiac murmur. That, associated with a plateau pulse and low blood pressure, made the diagnosis of a significantly tight aortic stenosis very likely. I was exceptionally impressed with my clinical acumen, as I was sure I was right. I did all the right medical things, referring him on etc. etc. and wrote a detailed letter to his general practitioner. A few days later, my boss collared me, asking if I had seen this man. Of course, I responded that I had and that he had a tight aortic stenosis and I had done this, that and the other. The boss said "did you ask what his job was?" "Ahhh" I thought, no. Well, it turned out that he was a steeple jack. He should never have been doing any exercise let alone being allowed to climb up a chimney as people did at that time without any safety harnesses. I ought to have put him on light duties.

Aortic stenosis is a tightening of the valve as blood leaves the heart, to go to the rest of the body. The amount of blood leaving his heart was dangerously low and he could have fainted or collapsed at any time, particularly following the sort of exertions that climbing up three hundred feet chimneys were likely to produce. I also came across an unfortunate suicide attempt by a psychiatrist. This really was a Machiavellian attempt, designed to ensure his death at the hands of his treating doctors. Basically, he had put drops in one eye to dilate the pupil and given himself a massive overdose of insulin, at which point, he fell to the floor. His fall was heard and an ambulance summoned. He arrived at the casualty department, comatose, with one dilated eye pupil and the other small. The combination of coma and pupil inequality following a fall would normally suggest some sort of intracranial haemorrhage, with extradural haemorrhage being highly likely, given the speed of onset. There were no MRI scans or CT scans. Under those suspicious circumstances, it would have been standard practice to have drilled four holes into the skull, two on each side, in the hope of locating the clot and releasing it. Had that been done without his low blood sugar being recognised and treated, he would certainly have died. Fortunately, a very astute senior physician picked up the slightly increased pulse rate and subtle sweating and gave him intravenous glucose without even checking the blood sugar. He came round virtually instantly.

I remember being in a clinic, assisting the boss who had students in tow. An older lady, who was significantly overweight, enquired as to whether her obesity could be glandular in nature. The boss, clearly wanting to show off in front of the students, said "well madam, I suppose it could be but only if you call your mouth a gland".

With another patient, he unfortunately made a particularly silly mistake, in retrospect. He told some overweight lady that she ought to be able to work out the cause, as nobody came out of Belsen her size. The grin on his face was wiped out instantly, when she burst into tears and showed him her Auschwitz tattoo.

Taking proper dietary histories can help to determine calorie intake but are best done by experienced dieticians (it is not dietitian – they are not "tits"). Doctors generally do this sort of enquiry badly. Once I saw a woman on a home visit who was 30 odd stones and morbidly obese.

She claimed to eat very little and started to describe a typical day's food intake. Breakfast was a bowl of cereal and milk, no toast, and a cup of tea – unremarkable. Before she could proceed further her friend hinted that I should see the bowl and sourced it from the kitchen. Her breakfast "bowl" was in fact a family sized casserole dish!

There is the tale of the young and innocent. Mrs Innocent was a young housewife with three daughters. The family pet white rabbit, Snowball, lived in style inhabiting a large hutch at the side of the house and having a "run" in the back garden. Late one afternoon their next-door neighbour Mrs Young heard a kerfuffle in her own back garden. The Young's boxer dog was leaping around and growling with Snowball in his jaws. Snowball was being violently shaken and intermittently dragged through the mud. Mrs Young managed to separate them and locked the dog in the garage. Snowball was filthy dirty, limp and clearly dead but there were no visible bite marks or bleeding. The evidence suggested that the dog had grabbed Snowball from either its "run" or hutch and killed it by snapping her neck whilst "worrying it". One of two simple choices had to be made. Go next door and confess at the earliest opportunity (the Innocents were out for the day) or obfuscate matters by leaving a false set of clues. She chose the latter. A large bowl of soapy water was run and Snowball washed clean and blow-dried with a hair dryer. Mrs Young sneaked next-door and placed the corpse of Snowball in a sleeping position back in the hutch. Snowball had obviously died peacefully in her sleep. "End of the matter"

Two days later Mrs Young answered a knock on her door to be confronted by the police making house-to-house enquiries. They were looking for a "sick pervert" causing nuisance. The circumstances were that Snowball had in reality died peacefully in her sleep, but some five days earlier. The Innocent family had held a burial service in the garden. Kind words had been spoken, tears shed, and flowers laid on the grave. The police were seeking the person who had deliberately caused the Innocents distress by disinterring Snowball and putting her back in the hutch.

A chronically ill patient died not unexpectedly on the ward just before the night staff came on duty. The male nurse on day duty ought to have dealt with the "last offices", paperwork and informed the next of kin. He was however in a rush to finish and came up with a plan. The "patient" was propped up comfortably on pillows and a hot cup of tea placed by the bedside to give the impression of life and well-being. Hand over was successfully accomplished and off he went. The night staff, realising what he must have done and being both busy and short-staffed, took no action other than to place another hot cup of tea beside him just before the offender returned for the next day's early shift!

Unnecessary delays in issuing death certificates distresses grieving relatives. The certifying doctor has to be one who has actively been treating the deceased within the last 28 days. Normally that is not a problem in hospital. However, change overs in August and February, especially if they coincided with annual leave, could occasionally produce the situation whereby no-one who fulfilled the criteria was still around if death happened in certain short periods with one doctor having left and his successor not yet having seen the patient. One Consultant had the simple solution. Before moving to the next job the juniors were told to write and sign the certificate for any likely deaths beforehand leaving just the date to be inserted as and when. Quick, simple solutions to complex problems are almost always wrong!

In the "good old days" schemes to legally avoid "death duties" depended as they still do on survival for seven years after the estate has been reduced. However, the current taper relief which applies reducing tax as the years pass was not introduced for some time. It was all or nothing – death within seven years attracted the full tax, death afterwards nothing. If deaths occurred at home a few days before the threshold, corpses could be hidden, kept cool and presented later to doctors as more recent deaths. Suspicious doctors could be put under considerable pressure to collude. One little known fact applicable today is that the estates of those who have died from wounds or other injuries suffered during military service for the monarch are exempt of all inheritance tax. To qualify, those injuries have to be a contributory cause which is more than trifling. Many lawyers have successfully argued that a gunshot wound many years earlier will have contributed to death. Few doctors are likely to say that having been shot years before has made someone healthier!

The Latin language completely foxed me and once I realised that it was not a required subject for medicine, we parted company. However, hand written on the flyleaf of my school Latin primer were the phrases "Latin is a language, as dead as dead could be. It killed the ancient romans and now it's killing me" and "Noli illegitimi carborundum" purporting to mean "Don't let the bastards grind you down." A motto which stayed with me. Around this time I learnt that, despite it sounding erudite, it was not Latin at all! It was made up and used in WW2 by the US General Stilwell as his motto. Latin scholars tell me that "Noli nothis permittere te terere" meaning "Don't let the bastards wear you down." Would be more correct, though it lacks the same punch.

CHAPTER FIVE

Gaining Seniority and Knowledge

The winter of 1978/79, became known as 'the winter of discontent', due to the large numbers of public service staff who went on strike. This had just come to an end at the time of my appointment as the Registrar to the Professorial Unit, based at Broadgreen Hospital. Broadgreen was situated at the eastern periphery of the city, close to the M62 motorway. It was walking distance from Knotty Ash, of Ken Dodd fame. Historically, it had been founded in the early 1900s as a TB sanatorium and had acquired a formidable reputation for the treatment of heart and lung conditions (in the early days, the treatment of TB was largely based on good food and fresh air). Beds were placed outdoors on covered verandas open to the elements to take advantage of the fresh air and sun. Surgical techniques had been developed in order to collapse and rest infected parts of the lung. By crushing the phrenic nerve in the neck, part of the diaphragm could be paralysed, causing collapse of the lower lung segments and by removing some ribs and allowing the chest wall to collapse, the top of the lung could also be rested. These treatments were undoubtedly lifesaving at the time but produced complications in later life. The bombing of Liverpool in WW 2 destroyed large parts of Mill Road Hospital and medical beds were hastily relocated to the Broadgreen site. These were emergency medical service wards, which were temporary single storey structures, connected by corridors but were still in use until the mid-1980's In essence, the site at Broadgreen was large, with the corridors being an 'H' shape, minus one of the limbs. It was a very friendly hospital and being single storey with long corridors, you frequently got to bump into staff on your meanderings. There was a busy traditional casualty department, which was the hub for most acute medicine.

Having acquired my full Membership, I was technically the senior of the registrars on site. As such, I was in charge of organising educational meetings, the rota and generally being the junior medical administrative 'dog's body'. I had the advantage of being parachuted into a fairly senior position, with most of my student antics and junior doctor errors being unknown. I had acquired a great deal of experience and felt confident taking up this role. The medical registrar is normally the most senior physician on site in a hospital at nights and weekends. Consultants were, of course, available for advice from home and/or would come in, if required. However, the routine work, dealing with acutely medically ill patients was 'bread and butter' stuff for a competent medical registrar. My first few nights on-call allowed me to establish a reputation for being efficient and competent, which smoothed my induction.

It took me a while to appreciate the legendary Liverpudlian humour. One patient, by the name of Keith

Miller, winked and introduced himself with the words "I'm the killer". This took me aback until I realised that it was the anagram of his name that had caused him to acquire the nickname 'Killer' in school. Thomas Andrew Hawk was universally known as 'Tomahawk.' One of the nurses, Ruth Safta – R Safta, was known as Heady, as she was reputed to always go head first. I was assured by a carpet fitter, who was a patient, that his main occupational hazard was 'getting felt up the back passage'. The Broadgreen casualty, at that time, was busy and somewhat dilapidated. The phone system was old-fashioned, being operated by ladies in the main switchboard who would respond to lights flashing by plugging in connections. There was no internal dialling system. To get an outside line, you merely picked up the phone until the switchboard operator answered and you requested an outside line or internal connection. The walls around the main phone in the nurses' office had key phone numbers scrawled thereon. On one particular night on-call, I needed to get hold of a psychiatrist at Rainhill Hospital. Next to the words 'Rainhill' was written a telephone number. I went through switchboard and asked them to connect me to that number. The phone rang out and was quickly answered with a voice saying "Ello mate", with a pause. In the background, I could hear a small baby squawking, a toddler shouting and a woman shrieking. I paused. I asked whether I had got through to Rainhill Hospital. There was a further pause and the voice replied "Well, no mate but it seems like it". It turned out that I had phoned some random number, probably an off-duty member of staff, and I certainly began to appreciate the subtle nature of the Liverpool humour. An old 'Docker', lying on his bed, breathing through an oxygen mask, during a ward round, mumbled the words "Are me testicles black"? I looked at him and then looked at the nurse at the other side of the bed, who shrugged her shoulders. I drew the curtains around, pulled down the bed cover and investigated. His testicles were not black. I reassured him. He then ripped off the oxygen mask and said "Are me test results back"? In those days, there was no such thing as evidence based medicine. Treatments were empirical and often based on whims and experience. There were very few guidelines in place. Even when guidelines for certain treatments came into being much later, experienced people appreciated that they were the guidance for wise men but not rules, which were for fools to obey. One very breathless man had severe acute heart failure. His lungs were filling with fluid and despite standard treatment via the mnemonic MADDOG (morphine, aminophylline, diuretics, digoxin, oxygen and god) he was worsening. The situation looked hopeless. A senior consultant with much experience gave him 20mls of intravenous brandy straight out of the ward stock bottle! He responded well to this unorthodox treatment which probably worked by reducing the "afterload" through vasodilation.

It is said that a physician is only as good as his knowledge of pathology. There was a long tradition at Broadgreen Hospital of performing post mortem examinations. Students and junior doctors normally attended and would be able to compare the pathology, to that which had been diagnosed on the basis of clinical examination and tests. There were some surprising findings. A man whose lung shadow had been presumed to be lung cancer, without biopsy, had received extensive radiotherapy treatment and as a result of this and recurrent pneumonias, had died. Post mortem examination revealed a large lung mass, centred upon a tiny foreign body that turned out to be a rabbit vertebra.

He had obviously inhaled this small bone during a meal and this set in train, an extensive localised infection, which had manifest itself as an enlarging lung shadow, and was completely misdiagnosed.

At that time, human growth hormone for treatment was being developed. Growth hormone is produced by the pituitary gland, situated just beneath the brain. It is a small pea sized gland. Pituitary glands were routinely harvested at post mortem examination and placed in large jars, containing some sort of preservative. A neighbouring hospital also participated. This was a traditional long-stay geriatric hospital and most of the patients therein were very elderly, frail and with a high incidence of dementia. Any that underwent post mortem also had their pituitary glands harvested. It would take some six months or so for the jar to be filled to capacity, with perhaps of the order of one thousand or more pituitary glands. Once full, they were collected by someone from the pharmaceutical industry and sent off for processing. The upshot was that growth hormone was extracted, purified and put into clinical use. Unfortunately, no-one knew the dangers. The infectious agent of CJD (mad cow disease) is a prion. These are said to be indestructible. It would only take a few prions in one of those pituitary glands to contaminate a huge batch and indeed, many of the recipients acquired CJD and died.

One of my roles was to organise the finals examination. This occurred within weeks of my starting. I had scoured the inpatient beds for patients with suitable histories and physical signs and had been given a list of phone numbers of patients who could come in from home. It was a fairly comprehensive list, the usual heart murmurs could be sourced; individuals with large kidneys, large spleens, funny neurological deficits and the usual chest conditions. The charge-nurse on the ward was highly experienced in running this show and we worked extremely well as a team. Beds were immaculately made; the 'patients' came into the ward, undressed and suitably lay on the bed, awaiting a succession of student examinations. One star patient was 'Claude'; an elderly man, with an impressively large spleen. He had attended for years as a short case. His profound deafness, only partially corrected by a hearing aid, made him unsuitable as a long case, as taking a history was very difficult. On the day in question, 'Claude' had failed to appear. We were depending on him. He was normally reliable; 8.00 am became 9.00 am and became 10.00 am and the examination was starting. No sign of 'Claude', until we had a phone call from the casualty department, asking if we were expecting 'Claude'? We all said "Yes" and 'Claude' was bundled up to the ward and put to lie on his designated bed. Students came and went. There was a short break for tea and biscuits and the examination resumed. The next student taken by a pair of examiners to examine 'Claude', found him unresponsive. He had in fact died.

The circumstances were somewhat tragic. 'Claude' had indeed been prepared to attend the examination. However, in the early hours of the morning, he had been taken ill at home. An ambulance had picked him up from home and taken him to casualty. Unfortunately, his inability to give a history had led to confusion. It was assumed that he was attending the examination and therefore not examined in the casualty department and merely dispatched up to the ward.

One of my patients was discharged home. She had been admitted with a number of falls and faints but was perfectly well at the time of discharge. I thought no more of it, until I received a phone call from the local police. I was apparently the last one to have seen her alive. She had been found at the bottom of her front garden, behind the hedge, with ante-mortem strangle marks around her neck. She was wet from a rain shower but the ground beneath was dry. It could be reasonably established that she had died within a relatively small window of time. I was asked whether she had strangulation marks on her neck at the time of discharge. I attended a post mortem and indeed, there were quite gross marks on either side of the neck, which could not have been missed, had she had them at the time of discharge. Murder was suspected but eventually excluded. What had happened was almost certainly this – she had arrived home without problem and had gone for a potter down her long front garden; she was leaning on her wooden picket gate fencing, watching the world go by. She must have had a collapse, which resulted in her neck being trapped between two of the narrow gate fencing staves. It was that which had produced the marks. She then must then have had a fit from lack of blood supply to the brain and in the course of the throws, flung herself sideways, behind the hedge. There was no other credible explanation and her death was considered to have been from natural causes.

Another of my patients was a very elderly man, who had an unusual claim to fame. As a young baby, he had been photographed sitting on the knee of an old man who had been a drummer boy at the battle of Waterloo. He said that this had always brought him good luck, which he wished to pass on. He touched my hand, such that I could claim that I had been touched on the hand by a man who had sat on the knee of a man who had been at the battle of Waterloo.

During the 1970s, and indeed until quite late into the 1980s, nurse training was very traditional. Students worked on the wards as essential pairs of hands, receiving their theoretical education in the classroom, in short blocks of study. Practical skills were taught on the wards by the ward staff, assisted by designated clinical tutors. One of my registrar roles was to give the occasional lectures to those in classrooms. Nurses traditionally either worked the early shift, starting before breakfast and finishing late afternoon, or the late shift, starting around lunch time and finishing at 9.00 pm. The actual hours of the night shift varied between hospitals but were roughly between 9.00 pm and breakfast time. As each shift changed, there was an overlap of some hours – far more than was needed to allow for hand over. Student nurses, surplus to requirements often received ad hoc teaching from the "medics".

It was not unusual for relatively junior first year student nurses to be left in charge of the wards for very short periods whilst the seniors took their breaks. Third year student nurses were often the most senior people actually on the wards at night. They were loosely supervised by night sisters, who routinely visited on "rounds" and were available in the event of some disaster. The giving of night sedation was fairly routine practice. One evening, a third year student nurse misread the prescription of Heminevrin 500 mg, as Heminevrin 500 ml. As alluded to earlier, when the dose of any liquid medication exceeds 10 ml, it is probably wrong. However, undaunted and not having access to a suitable 500 ml beaker, she sourced a pint beer glass from the doctors' mess. Into this, she decanted the entire ward stock contents of Heminevrin from her own ward and some from the stock bottles on adjacent wards. She estimated that if she almost filled the pint glass and then extracted some 60 ml, she would be left with roughly 500 ml. The patient was handed his medication at the bedside and over the course of half an hour, managed to consume the contents. He went to sleep and continued to sleep for a further forty-eight hours. There was a quiet "bollocking" given by the night sister but the patient was led to believe that he had a new sleep treatment being piloted on the ward.

On one busy night, a staff nurse from the casualty department was drafted onto the ward to man the phones, whilst the regular staff and the night sister dealt with a particularly sick patient. She received a phone call from a man, phoning from outside the hospital, enquiring about his father, who he had realised had been admitted. She mixed up the patients and wrongly told the man that his father was seriously ill. What she did not know was that the man was phoning from Australia. He immediately got the first plane home and arrived on the ward, tired and dishevelled, after a twenty-four hour flight, to find that his father was perfectly well. Two patients, John and Eddie, had been transferred in the same ambulance, to hospital, together. Eddie had had a below knee amputation. John had all four limbs intact. They were admitted to different wards. Unfortunately, their records, which had been transferred with them, got mixed up. John was asked by the admitting nurse if it was OK to call him Eddie, to which he answered yes. The absence of the amputation was not picked up by the admitting doctor and John proudly found himself in a bed with the label 'Eddie' above his head. He received all of Eddie's medication. He underwent x-rays, designed for Eddie. It took some three days before the mistake was realised. There was hell to pay. How could this mistake have happened? Quite simply, when John was asked whether he could be called Eddie he said yes because he didn't like the name John and always fancied being called Eddie!

Some drugs have similar sounding names and some have very similar spellings. If written in a hurried scrawl, mistakes in dispensing can result. Chlorpropamide is now a somewhat old fashioned oral hypoglycaemic drug, used to lower blood sugar and treat diabetes. Chlorpromazine was a major sedative, normally prescribed at night. At around midnight, on five successive nights, a patient on Chlorpromazine collapsed. He had the classic signs of a raised pulse and sweating, suggesting a low blood sugar. On each and every occasion, he responded to glucose. The rare condition insulinoma was suspected (natural insulin is produced by the beta cells of the islets of Langerhans, in the pancreas. These produce insulin in response to a raised blood sugar and switch off production as the blood sugar level falls. Those cells can develop tumours. Such tumours are under less bodily control than the normal cells and can produce large quantities of inappropriate insulin, leading to attacks of hypoglycaemia). The presence of an insulinoma was suspected here. Nowadays, it is a relatively easy condition to diagnose but then, much less so and occasionally involved exploratory abdominal surgery. Fortunately, before matters had gone that far, an astute nurse queried whether there had been a mix up between the prescribed Chlorpromazine and the actual Chlorpropamide which had been given. I presented this case at one of our clinical meetings. One of the senior physicians related a tale from his junior days. He had strongly suspected an insulinoma in a patient on his ward. He was a senior registrar and very experienced at the time. His then boss was more sceptical. The only way to solve that problem was to arrange for a surgeon to open the abdomen and do an exploratory operation. He was taken to one side by the boss, who said, "You go to theatre with the surgeon and if your diagnosis is wrong boy, pack your bags and go home, never to return". Fortunately, he was right.

As well as being responsible for teaching, I was also learning. One of the specialties which I learned was gastroenterology. I became adept at upper GI endoscopy and doing liver biopsies. An emergency gastroscopy was being done towards the end of the day within the gastroenterological unit, which was a separate building from the main hospital. The man was haemorrhaging and died of natural causes during the procedure. Technically, had correct procedure been followed, he ought to have been tidied up where he was and the body duly transferred to the mortuary. Staff were packing up after a long day and no one was willing to stay behind in the isolated building, with a corpse. It was decided that the greater good would be served by pretending that he was still alive. An oxygen mask was placed on his face and he was rushed down the corridor, back to his own bed. Unfortunately, his relatives were in the corridor, as we passed. We had to wait a decent interval, before informing them of his passing. The matron was not impressed, asking me whether I was in the regular habit of wheeling corpses around the corridors, willy-nilly. One young attractive nurse fancied one of the senior house officers. Their passion was aroused one afternoon and they disappeared into the linen room (linen rooms are infamous for this). They were caught in 'the act' by the ward sister. The fate of the nurse was that she was

104

sacked. The doctor suffered no such sanction. His seniors saw the humour in it and just warned him not to get caught again.

A recognised complication from liver biopsy is a small haemorrhage, which usually will settle spontaneously. Just occasionally, a haematoma can form just beneath the liver capsule, causing pain, discomfort and fainting. I had never met this complication. I must have been doing my hundredth liver biopsy when it happened to me. With needle in the patient's liver, accessed from the right hand side of the chest, the patient suddenly went pale, screamed out in pain and fainted back onto the bed. His pulse was rapid and thready and blood pressure low. These were potentially the signs of a catastrophic haemorrhage. I thought I might have hit an artery. I frantically tried to find a surgeon but the seniors were all in theatre. Fortunately, his pulse settled and blood pressure returned to normal within an hour.

One of the junior surgeons came to see one of our elderly ladies, who had a suspicious breast lump. He decided it would be appropriate to biopsy this on the ward, using one of the True-cut biopsy cutting needles normally used on the liver. The patient lay flat on her back, the breast was exposed, cleansed and the needle introduced. What happened next was shocking. Within seconds of the needle being inserted, the patient sat bolt upright and coughed a large amount of blood all over the place and died. What had happened was obvious, surely. In fact, two and two did not add up to four as post mortem examination confirmed. The needle had barely gone millimetres into the breast tissue and had gone nowhere near the lung or heart. She did however have an underlying condition called bronchiectasis and it had been a coincidence that at that moment she had haemorrhaged from it and died.

Where the ribs join the sternum, there are tiny joints, which can become inflamed. I saw one such case in the outpatient clinic. The patient was a robust looking middle age man, with a manual job and clearly in some discomfort. I thought I would solve this problem with a little steroid injection. The steroid and a local anaesthetic were drawn up and I carefully inserted a tiny needle into one of these small joints. As I injected, he collapsed. He had fainted from the short-lived but excruciating pain of my injection. He soon came round.

I came across patients who, in an earlier life, had unfortunately been prisoners of war, having been captured by the Japanese. These people had terrible experiences at the time and few fully recovered, being left with physical and mental sequelae. Many had acquired a tropical worm, called strongyloides, which had never been diagnosed or treated. It caused an intermittent rash periodically if small numbers of the worms migrated but patient and worm lived in relative symbiotic harmony. However, if the patients became immunosuppressed, the worms could start their travels around the body in large numbers and cause serious problems including death. If diagnosed, treatment was simple and effective. The Liverpool School of Tropical Medicine took the lead in contacting old soldiers, screening and treating. I learned fairly rapidly to be very cautious about giving any immunosuppressant drugs, such as steroids, to anyone who had been in the Far East. One patient always attended carrying an old chest x-ray to prove the futility of doing further x-rays – his chest wall was full of fine shrapnel dust which prevented most of his lung from being visible.

The common antiemetic, Maxolon, has a rare but unusual side effect. It basically can cause an extrapyramidal reaction with torticollis. The neck of a patient can go into spasm, with a peculiar twist. If correctly diagnosed, it can be reversed in seconds by an injection of benztropine mesylate. One such case appeared in casualty, whilst I had students in tow. I could not resist impressing them with my diagnostic acumen and made a great show of how I was going to cure this man within thirty seconds. The patient was relieved and the students gathered around. The needle was inserted and injection given. I was a hostage to fortune. They started to count, slowly, 28, 29, 30, 31 – no response to my injection – smiles at my misfortune started to emerge on the faces of students, aware of my discomfort – 32, 33, 34, 35 – beaming smirks were now visible – 36, 37, 38, 39, 40. By now, the patient was disconcerted. Fortunately, when we reached 42, there was an instant cure.

A patient who had suffered some brain damage from a stroke was most distressed. He was lying in bed, mumbling "Feed me, feed me". He suddenly had a cardiac arrest and died. As this was unexpected, a post mortem was performed and the cause of death established. A clue had been given from a conversation given by a mobile man with dementia, who had approached the ward sister, volunteering the information that he had 'only given him a banana'. In fact, what had happened was to appease the shouts of 'feed me'; the man with dementia had unzipped a banana and pushed it into his mouth, such that it went straight into the trachea, causing his cardiac arrest and death. Post mortem revealed that his trachea was completely occluded with a relatively whole peeled banana.

Iripta Bolokov was an elderly Russian fairground strong man/wrestler. He was well over six feet tall and all muscle and bone. His forearms were the size of my thigh. You shook his hand at your peril. His party-trick on the ward was to cut an apple in two, having placed it between his fingers and chopping it with a scissor-like action. He could also do it with walnuts. He was also an expert on the 'hallucinogenic magic mushrooms'. The magic mushroom amanita muscarina contains the toxins muscarine and psilocybin. He claimed that to enjoy the hallucinogenic benefits without the accompanying vomiting and visual disturbance from pupil widening, the traditional Siberian trick was to feed the caps to the women and then drink their urine, while they were off being sick. He reckoned that the Laplanders would feed the mushroom caps to the reindeer and drink the reindeer urine. Whether or not this explains the term 'getting pissed', I know not.

Another educated man enthralled the junior nurses one afternoon by catching flies. The fly was approached with two handkerchiefs, one in each hand, from opposite directions. Apparently, its instinct to any threat, being programmed by its compound eye and nervous system, is for it to fly off in the opposite direction. By approaching with handkerchiefs from two directions, it confused it and it remained stationary, being easily picked up.

An academic economist we had in as a patient for tests had recently returned from New York and had been introduced to the new Tax theory which we now know as "The Laffer Curve" He was not ill and became bored as an in-patient. As such he gave an impromptu lecture on this at one of our medical meetings.

The Laffer Curve can be seen on the Laffer Centre web site http://www.laffercenter.com

The Laffer Curve is a skewed, vaguely bell shaped/ parabolic graph obtained by plotting the income tax rates levied against the total tax revenues actually collected by the government.

At a tax rate of 0%, the government would collect nothing, just as it would collect no tax revenue at a tax rate of 100% because it is unlikely that anyone would be willing to work for no take-home pay. Tax rates have two effects on revenues due to the interplay between the basic arithmetic and wider economic issues. The arithmetical effect itself theoretically ought to be predictable with a linear rise or fall in revenue proportional to the rise or fall in the tax rate. Put simply if a 1% tax collects £1 million, then people might assume that a 2% tax would collect £2 million...and so on.

However, the science of economics recognises that tax rates influence the motivation to work and earn money. When individuals, with reasonable incomes, realise that high tax rates penalise further earnings they become progressively disinclined to work and earn more. The tipping point and top of the "bell" is around the 50% tax rate. Thus, the Laffer Curve neatly demonstrates what happens when the economic and arithmetic effects of a tax rise or fall interact, explaining why a tax increase may reduce earnings and raise less revenue than otherwise predicted, just as a tax cut may increase taxed activity and raise more revenue than otherwise predicted.

The Laffer Curve apparently earned its name from a 1978 article by the late Jude Wanniski entitled, "Taxes,

Revenues, and the 'Laffer Curve." Wanniski recalled a 1974 dinner he attended with Arthur Laffer (Professor at The University of Chicago), Donald Rumsfeld (chief of staff to President Gerald Ford), and Dick Cheney (Rumsfeld's deputy and a former classmate of Laffer's). When the foursome's dinner discussion turned to President Ford's "WIN" (Whip Inflation Now) proposal for tax increases, Dr Laffer is said to have grabbed his napkin to sketch the curve as an illustration of the trade-off between tax rates and tax revenues. Wanniski dubbed the trade-off described as the "Laffer Curve." Although the Laffer Curve bears his name, the ideas behind it were not new or his alone. In fact, Dr Laffer himself liked to point out that the idea was so straightforward that people knew about it hundreds of years before. The Muslim philosopher, Ibn Khaldun, wrote in the 14th century that during the ruling dynasty of the time the revenues fell. At the beginning of the dynasty, taxation yielded large revenue from small tax rates. At the end of the dynasty, taxation yielded smaller revenues even though the tax rates had risen.

Whenever governments introduce new taxes, they have unintended consequences owing to tax avoidance strategies. The window tax (repealed in 1851) led to windows being bricked up. The tax on individual bricks (1784-1850) was avoided as the number of bricks used in building a house decreased when manufacturers increased their size. Houses in Amsterdam were taxed according to their width resulting in the tall narrow houses.

The law of unintended consequences applies to other fields including the pharmaceutical industry. Many "wonder drugs" have come and gone. Indomethacin is a well-established anti-inflammatory drug used in arthritis.

It is however highly irritant to the lining of the stomach and gut causing ulceration occasionally leading to perforation and peritonitis. To circumvent this and to attempt to deliver a steady dose the preparation "Osmosin" was invented. The indomethacin was contained within an insoluble plastic capsule into which a single small hole was drilled by laser. The idea was that the capsule would slowly release the drug during its passage through the gut achieving steady blood levels without irritating the intestinal lining. It was heavily promoted as being safe and effective until there was a rise in small bowel perforation and peritonitis. The preparation was withdrawn in 1983 when it was realised that if the capsule lodged in the folds of the lining of the small bowel the pinpoint release of Indomethacin through the laser hole would simply drill a hole through the gut wall. The cholesterol lowering drug, Clofibrate, was withdrawn when it became apparent that deaths from "all causes" rose in those taking it. The reason has never been established. Eusol, (Edinburgh University solution of lime – chlorinated lime and boric acid) basically a mild bleach was a popular and very effective antiseptic dressing for wounds especially leg ulcers. Concern that it destroyed granulation tissue and delayed healing led to its withdrawal in the 1990's. That was followed by a rise in MRSA wound contamination.

The simple rule, 'I before E, except after C' does not work for a lot of the time. It does however work if the full rule is recited. This is 'I is before E, except after C, if the vowel sound rhymes with the word bee'. It does not therefore apply to words like deign or reign but is correct for almost all words except protein, seize and caffeine.

As my two years at Broadgreen Hospital came to a close, I needed to look for further positions. For a while, I had fancied gastroenterology but realised that I did not want to be so specialised in the future. What I liked, above all, was general medicine, which was a specialty in decline. The alternative and best mix for me was geriatric medicine. It provided the variety of conditions and the opportunity to meet fascinating individuals along the way. At that time, arrogant physicians maintained that geriatricians were those unfit to be let loose on patients who mattered. So, my choice of this specialty was viewed with some suspicion by my general physician peers. Nonetheless, I secured a post of senior registrar in geriatric medicine and spent the ensuing trainee period between the Royal Liverpool Hospital, under the Professor and Newsham General.

Newsham General was not a general hospital. Its roots were as a poor law workhouse. The standards of nursing care, however, were exceptionally high despite the facilities for the most part being poor. Some newer wards had been built, which provided facilities suitable for the admission of acutely ill patients. There was no casualty department on site; patients could be admitted directly into the receiving room, at the request of general practitioners or from the Broadgreen Hospital casualty department (now called A&E), if they were elderly and deemed suitable and fit enough for transfer. Thus began my career in geriatric medicine. Medical illness in old people is interesting and commonly treatable with beneficial results. The elderly remain amongst the most grateful patients of all.

CHAPTER SIX

People, Places and Oddities

Geriatric medicine is complex medicine: it is unusual to deal with a single disease entity. Geriatricians routinely deal with multiple pathology and the complicated interplay between impairment, disability and handicap. A geriatric patient is one who is lucky enough to be under the care of a geriatrician. Impairment simply refers to the reduction in a function of part of the body. Disability refers to the way in which impairment affects the function of an individual. Handicap is a term used to refer to the way in which impairment and disability affect a patient's resettlement back into their home/community. Taking a simple example of a left-handed lady with left elbow/forearm weakness, matters can be illustrated as follows. Her impairment is restricted movement of the left elbow and forearm. If she were otherwise well, her disability would be limited to lifting heavy objects with the left hand and perhaps writing. However, if she also had arthritis of her knees and required a walking aid, which the impairment of the left arm precluded, then her disability would also include the inability to walk. Her resultant handicap would depend upon her home environment. If she lived on the ground floor, with easy wheelchair access, her handicap could be minimised by the provision of an electric wheelchair. However, if her environment was only accessible by steps or she had stairs at home, she would be seriously handicapped and would probably have to move house.

Old age is not for 'sissies'. Sadly, it is accompanied by the gradual loss of sensation and mobility and the advent of successive impairments. In essence, the point is reached where things are taken from you. The list is endless but loss of teeth, hair, clarity of sight, clarity of hearing, strength and vigour are bad enough but if added to that is loss of your thought process from dementia, life can be fairly miserable. One person is diagnosed with Alzheimer's disease every 15 minutes – it's a good job he can't remember it!

Many housebound elderly people are lonely. This can be felt particularly acutely around Christmas. It is not necessarily Christmas day itself, but the week or so before and after, when everyone else is busy. One pensioner in Norwich attracted attention by fastening a crucified Father Christmas to the front of his house. This so offended people that the police insisted he took it down. A Christmas Midnight Mass, doubtless fuelled by alcohol, generated into a mass brawl at a Catholic church in Southampton. A Christmas "elf" caught selling mistletoe on the streets of Eastbourne without a licence, was fought to the floor by police using pepper spray and batons when he refused to give his details and move on. One man bought an antique wooden artificial leg in a salesroom, wrapped it and gave it to his wife for Christmas labelled as "just a little stocking filler". She was not amused.

The Dutch have an unusual Christmas tradition where the Dutch Father Christmas, who is white, is traditionally accompanied by servants, who wear black makeup, curly wigs and large painted red lips. Dutch people deny that the tradition is racist and claim that the black faces originate from chimney soot. I once saw a grotesque picture of an evil looking Santa Claus, in a Kitchener pose, pointing a finger, under which was the legend 'I want you to spend a lot of money, to prove you love your family'. Here is a list of things that you can only get away with saying, at Christmas time:

- Would madam like stuffing?

- I prefer breast, to legs.

- Tying the legs together keeps the inside moist.

- Smother the butter all over the breasts.

- If I don't undo my trousers, I will burst.

- I have never seen a better spread.

- I'm in the mood for a little dark meat.

- Are you ready for seconds yet?

- It's a little dry; do you still want to eat it?

- Just wait your turn, you will get some.

- Don't play with your meat.

- Stuff it up between the legs, as far as it will go.

- Do you think you will be able to handle all these people at once?

- I don't expect everyone to come at the same time.

- You still have a little bit on your chin.

- How long will it take after you put it in?

- You'll know it's ready when it pops up.

- Just pull the end and wait for the bang.

- That's the biggest bird I've ever had.

- I'm so full, I've been gobbling nuts all morning.

- Wow, I didn't think I could handle all that and still want more.

- I do like a good stuffing.

Most people have heard of Rudolph the red nose reindeer but not everyone has heard of Bruno the brown nose reindeer. He allegedly rides behind Rudolph, but is not quite so quick at stopping.

The school Nativity play is a regular ritual, which occupies teachers and pupils in junior schools for weeks in the run-up to Christmas. It fuels excitement and expectation. Casting is traditional. A pretty little girl is chosen to be 'Mary', the class Adonis is chosen to be 'Joseph' and invariably, the Inn Keeper is played by somebody fat. The rest dress as various animals and those with access to gaudy tea towels come dressed as shepherds. One I attended went horribly wrong, when the lines were forgotten. Joseph and Mary knocked on the Inn Keeper's door, which the Innkeeper opened. They requested a room at the inn. The Innkeeper replied there was no room at the inn. It was here the record stuck. Joseph requested a room at the inn; the Innkeeper replied there was no room. This was repeated three or four times, before the Innkeeper burst into tears and said 'There's no room and it's not my fault'. Joseph's response was 'Well, if you read the book Pal, it aint mine either'. You can now count the number of days till Christmas.

When I started in geriatric medicine, it was suggested that I read Gulliver's Travels, particularly part three, chapter ten. This perceptive work, written by Jonathon Swift in 1727 is worth reading in its entirety. Thackeray observed that "It is a most moving discourse upon the miseries which would attend on human life if protracted beyond the ordinary period assigned to man". Basically, Gulliver came across the Luggnaggians and those amongst their number with a genetic abnormality were known as the Struldbrugs.

The Struldbrugs had a rare abnormality, which could turn up in any family at random. They were born with a red spot on their forehead, which signified immortality. The spot changed to green at puberty, blue at the age of twenty-five years and coal black at the age of forty-five. It never changed thereafter. The advantages of the gift of immortality were perceived as a lengthy life in order to procure riches. This was a time to excel at learning; a time to contemplate, observe and gain knowledge and wisdom and a lengthy life to witness the unfolding discoveries of science and the opportunity to use one's long life to reflect, audit and re-audit achievements. However, the gift of immortality was not associated with youth, health and vigour. In reality, the first thirty to forty years were normal but thereafter, they became increasingly melancholy and dejected, until they reached the normal maximum life expectancy of eighty years. By that time, they had collected the follies and infirmities of old age, together with all the extra negatives, which arose from the prospect of never dying. Their envy of youth and vigour was directed against the vices of the young and the deaths of the old. The least miserable were the ones with dementia, who were oblivious to their plight. The diseases, to which they were subject, continued their course. The changing nature of language led to problems with communication, such that they became like foreigners in their own land. Legal solutions had to be devised. Should two Struldbrugs' marry, the law automatically dissolved the marriage when the youngest reached the age of eighty years. It was felt that no one should have to have their miseries doubled by the presence of a spouse for that duration. To counteract the consequences of the greed of age, which would lead to Struldbrugs accumulating wealth and eventually owning the nation, they were considered to be dead-in-law after the age of eighty. As a consequence, their heirs inherited and only a small state pittance was provided.

Dealing with the elderly, I came across conditions which were otherwise rare. Dramatic and sometimes frightening hallucinations occur in those with poor eyesight. This is known as the Charles Bonnet syndrome. The hallucinations arise from the lack of stimulation of the visual cortex of the brain and are sometimes called release hallucinations, as they are released within the visual cortex to compensate for the absence of normal visual input from the outer world. They can be extremely vivid, featuring people in bright clothes, as well as animals, trees and houses. They last a few seconds before fading away and being replaced by others. Most people rationalise that they are transient but nonetheless, it can be distressing. Some patients think that they have seen ghosts, whereas, others keep quiet in case they may be institutionalised for being 'mad'.

Walking aids are frequently used, the most common being the walking stick. Such sticks are normally self-prescribed, rarely fit for purpose and used wrongly. Many people will use either a random stick, purchased in a shop, or one inherited from a long-deceased relative. The rules for using a stick are simple and I shall share the secret, in order to guarantee the reader endless hours of fun at airports, watching those who feign limps and disabilities, in order to ensure early boarding and better seats on the plane. Firstly, the stick ought to be held with the arm bent and used on the opposite side of leg disability. The body stance ought to be erect and the gait as fast as is comfortable. If so used, the stick provides stability. A stick is not a crutch and those who do not need a stick can be readily identified. They use a stick that is too short and hold it with a straight arm, on the side of the feigned leg disability. Stick and leg move together with a slow gait exaggerating any disability.

Rathbone hospital, where we had rehabilitation beds, held a fund-raising garden party each year. I went along with my three small daughters, all neatly dressed. We had been to the park in the morning to walk the dog and I had taken a walking stick with me, not really for use but more to fend off nuisance dogs. The youngest daughter had picked up a small stick in the park and copied my actions. When we arrived at the garden party, there were various stalls set up and I made a handful of purchases. On one of the tables was a walking stick and my youngest daughter wanted it. I asked one of the ward sisters, who was running the stall, how much she wanted for the stick. The price was duly agreed and I acquired the stick. It was clearly too large for a four-year-old but I sized it up, whipped out my Swiss army knife and sawed off some six inches and put the rubber ferule back on the end. She greeted me with a beaming smile and started to brandish the stick. At that moment, an elderly lady was heard to shout "Whose nicked me stick, I only rested it there for five minutes while I was looking at the stalls"? The stick had to be hastily hidden and we beat a smart retreat. One of the cruellest fates is to be both blind and deaf and live in a dark, silent world. We had one such patient on the ward. His few pleasures were eating and drinking but he appreciated conversations with sign language written on his palm. His sense of time was poor. In the early hours of one morning, a noisy man with dementia was disrupting the ward. The nurses had placed him in a wheelchair, in the empty day room, to minimise distress to others and in the hope that he would calm down with the absence of stimulation. My blind, deaf man awoke at about 6 am and was attended to by the nurses, who wheeled him in to the day room. The demented man woke up and started to shout towards my man and make gestures. My man was oblivious and made no response. The demented man became increasingly frustrated and this culminated in him picking up large heavy dinner plates from a stack and hurling them, discus style, across the room. One of them connected with the side of my man's head, knocking him out instantly. Within hours, he was dead. He had developed an extradural haematoma. The inside of the skull is lined by the dural membrane. Between that membrane and the skull are some small arteries. If they rupture from trauma, a significant amount of blood can accumulate directly underneath the skull and squash the brain below. Deterioration to the point off death can take a very short period. This is in contrast to subdural haemorrhage, which is normally a venous ooze between the dura and the brain. Whilst large clots can indeed develop, because the bleeding is at the rate of a venous ooze, rather than arterial blood pressure, it takes a lot longer. The cause of death was identified at a coroner's post mortem but no police action was taken, as the culprit clearly lacked any capacity. One patient had been an airline pilot. He had previously been in the RAF and retained a mischievous humour. After a successful flight, he would emerge from the cockpit in his uniform, wearing dark glasses and would tap his way down the aisle with a white stick. The passengers had clearly arrived safely and were not usually upset. He then changed tack. He would get on the plane with his uniform hidden under a scruffy mac. He would sit in an empty seat towards the back of the plane and stay quiet as the passengers boarded. He would then make lots of tut, tutting noises about the plane being late and where was the pilot etc. He would become increasingly noisy and then would jump up and say "If that pilot doesn't come soon, I'm going to fly it myself" and then would stride down the aisle and enter the cockpit. Of course, the stewardesses were in on the act but did not let on until there was a suitable amount of anxiety.

One mortuary technician, who had worked in some large central mortuaries, would like to tell the story about the police sergeant who used to initiate new constables in how to identify bodies. His trick was to climb into the fridge a few minutes before the constable would be coming and place himself perfectly still, under a white sheet, pretending to be a corpse. The moment the constable opened the fridge door he would of course sit up, making appropriate ghoulish sounds. This had been going on for a while before it was decided that he needed teaching a lesson. Just before he was about to play his part, someone else got in there first. The sergeant, duly arrived, crept in, put himself under the sheet and the door was shut. In the pitch dark, the sergeant heard a voice next door whispering "Eh, it's a bit cold in here isn't it". He never repeated his trick.

As a general rule, safety first is a good maxim. However, life is all about risk taking and this applies very much to the discharge of elderly patients back home. There will always be risks but the alternatives are to consign people to institutionalisation far too early. One sad case involved an elderly lady whose desire to return home was respected. She lived in a small cottage and spent much of her day sitting in an armchair, close to the hearth. She was supported by friends and neighbours and a home help went in most days. Sadly, she was found dead one morning, seemingly having rolled head first into the open fire, whilst trying to get up from the chair. Half her skull had been burned away.

Another man with mild confusion was thought to be safe to return home, having had an occupational therapist assess him, both in hospital and on a home visit. Sadly, he managed to burn his house down and risked the lives of his neighbours.

Many of our junior doctors had qualified overseas and had led somewhat colourful lives before coming to the UK. One of their number was Iranian, who had been based in Tehran during the Iraq/Iran war. He had been peacefully minding his own business at home, when he was awoken from sleep at 4.00 am, by an army detail, commanded by a captain. His name was 'on the list'. He was ordered to dress and escorted to the main square, to be met by the sight of over a hundred people tied to stakes awaiting execution. As the doctor on the 'list' his task was to replenish the blood banks at the front by bleeding each of these people of three to four pints of blood prior to their deaths.

Another junior doctor had been in the Iraqi forces, at roughly the same time. He assured me that it was standard practice to remove the kidneys from anyone executed, for sale/transplantation.

It may surprise you to know that the average number of legs per person is less than two. Apparently, the favourite ploy of an actuary was to wager that the next person to come through the door would have greater than the average number of legs. This is simply because of the prevalence of amputation. After an above knee amputation and as a general rule of thumb, the energy expended to walk a given distance is an extra 80% of that normally required. It is only an extra 40% for below knee amputees. Most amputations that are necessary in the elderly are the result of arterial disease. Arterial disease may manifest itself firstly in the legs but is usually associated with more widespread disease and general ill health. Not all do well. By contrast, traumatic amputations in the young and fit are normally associated with a reasonable degree of functional recovery. I was once on a TA exercise and the officer contingent was set the task of a fifteen kilometre forced march. This was across some fairly rough terrain. The ages of those in our group varied and there were a couple of colonels in their fifties. The younger element were eager to hare on ahead but the two colonels kept going at a decent steady pace and reached their destination without mishap. One of them had a commission in a Highland Regiment and he came to dinner, wearing his kilt. What did surprise us was that he had covered that distance at fair pace, having had a below knee amputation, many years before. One of the surgeons I was attached to as a student was an arterial surgeon who specialised in vascular reconstruction. Unfortunately, these would sometimes fail, leading to amputation. He knew his patients well and his party trick, to keep the students awake and attentive in outpatients, was to sit patients down, take their stick from them and whack the lower limb with a resounding bang. He used to do this regularly, until the inevitable happened. He had his patients mixed up and hit some poor old lady's normal right leg instead, by mistake. Although she was left with quite considerable bruising, she laughed it off. During the early 1980s, there were plenty of world war one veterans, still alive and reasonably healthy. War wounds at that time could easily be infected from the dirty uniforms and mud containing bacteria and tetanus spores. Antibiotics had not been discovered and amputation was often the only way to save lives. One of my patients had had an almost miraculous escape. He had been a machine gun casualty, who had got tangled up on the barbed wire in no-man's land and had remained there well into the night. A German patrol, who were repairing damaged barbed wire, found him. They provided some first aid, put him on a stretcher and took him back with them to their dug-out. His right lower leg was apparently in a terrible mess and he vividly recounted the story of being plied with Schnapps, before their infantry officer hacked off his leg as quickly as possible with a sword. The wound was sterilised with iodine and caulked with hot pitch. He was hospitalised in due course, became a prisoner of war and was ultimately repatriated as part of the Red Cross exchange, through Switzerland. His German issue prosthesis was still fully functional 60 years later and he had held down a manual job all his life. Another veteran had survived a cavalry sabre attack, which had opened his chest and abdomen before embedding itself in his thigh. He had lost the leg but made a fair recovery otherwise. Another man, a D-day veteran, shrugged off the fact that when his tank was hit, he was blown out and his left leg was left inside. Another of my patients with an amputated thumb, owed his life to Captain Noel Chavasse, VC and Bar. Captain Chavasse was awarded his first VC for bravery in Guillemont in August 1916, when he tended wounded men all day, under heavy fire and then searched for other injured soldiers at night, in front of the enemy lines. My patient was involved in the Passchendaele offensive of the summer of 1917, and whilst advancing, received a hand wound with partial amputation of his thumb on the left hand. He made his way to a first aid post, which had been set up in a captured German block-house. The door, which had once faced to the rear when it had been part of the German trenches, was now facing the enemy. Chavasse tended the wound, completed the amputation of the thumb and applied a bandage. My patient was not deemed ill enough to be evacuated but was sent back to the front. As he trudged reluctantly back to join his comrades, a shell flew overhead, entered the door and caused Chavasse's mortal wound. Almost certainly, had my man not been sent back up the line and stayed in the block-house he would have died. He told me of the three casualty clearing stations, Mendinghem, Dozinghem and Bandaghem. However, I am not sure whether he was telling the truth because they seem to sound suspiciously like 'Mending them, Dosing them and Bandage them' despite looking like proper Belgian place names.

There are, however, real place names which can raise a chuckle. The Amish town of Intercourse; Condom in France and Climax in Colorado are well-known. Iron knob in Queensland; Muff in Northern Ireland, Thong in Kent, Ugley in Essex and Dyckesville Wisconsin are less so. Brown Willy stands erect on Bodmin Moor. Many a lad has been roused passing by Wetwang on the A166 between York and Bridlington. Travelling south on the A483 near Oswestry the village of Knockin is sign posted. Before you have had time to wonder whether it has a shop you come to Pant! As a youth, I explored petting, being unaware of its existence as a place. Petting in Bavaria is where some travelling couples prefer to stop before going any further. Some go onto Wankum in Northwest Germany but it is quicker to press onto f***ing. The place of f***ing is a tiny hamlet in Austria (population 130) 33Km north of Salzburg, just to the east of the border with Germany. Dating back to before the 10th Century, it acquired its name from a minor noble, Focko, and prior to 1760 it was spelled as Fugkhing. Thereafter it received its current spelling identical to the word in English. It is a rural community with fresh air, lakes, forests and beautiful scenery. Virtually crimeless for centuries, the perennial theft of road signs became a problem after it came to the notice of American GI's stationed nearby. British troops soon started visiting to have their photographs taken. The signs as one enters the village have been rendered theft-proof after the police became fed up with the f***ing signs constantly being stolen. It is a popular spot for British tourists to dip into for a f***ing photo shoot. The locals love their f***ing community and cannot really understand the British obsession with their peaceful f***ing. They have refused to capitalise upon matters. There are no f***ing postcards and no T-shirts emblazoned with the slogan "I love f***ing in Austria".

There is a story about the Imperial Camel Corps which served with distinction in WW1 in Palestine and Egypt. It has been described as a collection of aristocrats and complete ruffians. The tale is told of one of their officers asking for a volunteer bugler. A particularly unsavoury character stepped forward. When he was quizzed about his talents, he apologised, having been under the misapprehension that it was a burglar that was wanted. A camel is of course a racehorse designed by a committee!

The term 'doolally' is a term used to describe somebody who is confused and muddled. There is a belief that this term originated from Doolally army transit camp, somewhere in India. Transit camps are pretty soul destroying places with few home comforts and little to do. Enduring the boredom, heat and flies was said to send you doolally.

Most parents tell their children that only boring people get bored. There may however be a scientific reason. It is thought that people with defective dopamine receptors are the ones who get bored more frequently than others. Dopamine is the neurotransmitter that produces the sense of joy and excitement in the brain. When levels drop, time seems to slow and life loses its savour. Dopamine levels are stimulated by excitement and particularly by risk-taking behaviours, ranging from bungee jumping, gambling, adultery and drink. The traditional remedy for boredom in small children is to give them a disagreeable job, such as weeding a flower bed or cleaning silver. Some respond to being told that boredom is a sign of low intelligence. I personally find that bored small children can be put to good use dusting skirting boards, especially as we know longer have chimneys which need sweeping.

Winston Churchill was allegedly sat next to an Air Chief Marshal's wife, who wore an aeroplane brooch on her ample chest. Noticing him looking at it, she enquired as to whether he was admiring her aeroplane. His response was apparently 'no madam, the aerodrome'.

An old sailor told me the story of the fog flag, which was flown from the signal station at Portsmouth. This was run up the yard-arm to warn mariners that it was foggy in the harbour. When the fog lifted and the flag could actually be seen, it was then taken down.

The phrase, cold enough to freeze the balls off a brass monkey, has naval origins. The brass monkey was the triangle upon which the cannon balls were stacked in a pyramid. In the cold the brass would contract more than the iron in the cannon balls and they would be squeezed off. I have often thought that a mini version for the garden would be a novel gift for Xmas. The recipient, after a very cold night, could truly comment upon the brass monkey weather!

These days, smoking is generally considered to be the single most preventable cause of premature death. It is now the ultimate out-door pursuit! Some people are more resistant to the harmful effects than others. It is estimated that every four cigarettes smoked takes an hour off your lifespan. On that basis, a twenty-a-day smoker, consuming eight thousand cigarettes per year, would, over a fifty-year smoking history, consume four hundred thousand cigarettes and lose one hundred thousand hours of life expectancy, which is about eleven and a half years.

Susceptibility to damage from alcohol is probably more varied but some regularly consume far in excess of the Government limits, without much evidence of harm.

Forty years of random casual sex, at a frequency of four times per week, would lead to some potential eight thousand exposures to sexually transmitted diseases.

Putting matters into perspective, one bullet, one rocket, one bayonet or one grenade could well prove lethal. I wonder which I would ban first if I was in government, smoking, drinking, sex, or war?

I heard the story of the American lady, Gertrude Janeway, who died in 2003 at the age of ninety-three years. At the age of eighteen she had escaped poverty by marrying an eighty-one-year-old man who was a veteran of the American civil war, having fought for the union forces. After he died, she was entitled to a lifelong civil war army pension.

There is a theory as to why most men are right handed. Left handers expose their left chest and heart when raising their sword arm and are more likely to die in battle. They may not breed and pass on their genetics. Lethal genetic conditions, such as sickle cell anaemia and cystic fibrosis, are only lethal when two genes are inherited. Carriers with only one gene are, by and large, minimally affected under normal circumstances but some sickling can occur under adverse circumstances. The carrier frequency for these conditions is surprisingly high. It is speculated that carriers of cystic fibrosis may have been historically protected against lethal diarrhoeal illness and those with a sickle cell trait may have been more resistant to malaria.

Afro-Caribbeans are more susceptible to a type of hypertension, which responds poorly to current medications. One theory is that their ancestors were much better at conserving sodium and water and as a consequence, were more likely to survive being enslaved in Africa and transported across the Atlantic. Those with that trait were more likely to arrive in a healthy state, breed and pass it on thus predisposing future generations to high blood pressure.

The signs of the well-being of the economy in general are all around. Shortages of taxis with cranes visible everywhere are signs of boom. Beggars and buskers in abundance signal the converse. The "Hot Waitress Index" is a joking variant on this theme. It suggests that as the economy improves, good-looking women get better and better work moving to the "pretty girl" jobs as receptionists and suchlike. They move to waitressing when times are harder.

A local supermarket had a children's ride outside, with the sign:

- Place child on ride.

- Insert coin in slot.

- Stand well back.

The general advice 'Give a man a fish and feed him for a day, teach a man to fish and you will have fed him for life' ought better to read 'Give a man a fish and feed him for a day, teach a man to fish and he will sit in a boat and drink beer all day'. It is alleged that fishing is better than making love. When you fish and you catch something, you are delighted. When you make love and catch something...

Locally, laminated wooden floors are referred to as "lesbian floors" because there are no nuts or screws – it's all tongue and groove.

CHAPTER SEVEN

Home Visiting

The visiting of patients at home by consultants, normally in the company of their general practitioner, has a long history antedating the establishment of the NHS. The NHS incorporated this practice and these formal domiciliary visits attracted an additional payment to consultants, reflecting roughly an hour and a half of salary, to take into account travel time etc. They were popularly requested from consultants in many specialties but by the 1980s, had become almost exclusively the domain of old age psychiatrists and geriatricians. They provide a wonderful insight into the lives of patients. Conflicting schedules led to it being progressively unusual for the general practitioner to actually attend. They are now rarely requested and very few are done. Over some 30 years, I performed over eight thousand such visits. The vast majority were unremarkable but a small percentage provided an insight into the bizarre and the macabre.

I was initiated into the basic rules and these are quite simple:

• Where possible, arrange to do the visit during the daylight. Elderly people living alone are generally reluctant to open the doors to strangers at night.

• Always park your car in such a way as to facilitate a quick getaway. It is almost impossible to get away from concerned relatives if you have to do a three point turn in a narrow side street with people continuing their conversations through the car window. On the other hand, a quick 'cheerio', start of the car and off, presents no problem.

• The gutters of small side streets are often littered with nails and screws, shed from the vans of jobbing builders. Beware.

• Always arrange for the dog to be put into the garden. In my experience, it is the small yappy dogs, which are the greatest menace.

• Always keep a can of insecticide spray in the car. If prophylactically applied to trouser bottoms and socks, fleas will be thwarted.

• Don't be afraid of visiting dodgy areas. Dubious characters with vicious dogs on leads lurking by the house you are due to visit are likely to be there for your protection.

• Beware of sitting in certain houses – you will recognise them quickly. Try to avoid accepting cups of tea and never accept nibbles or biscuits. Biscuit barrels can be full of ants and nuts may not be quite what you think (one old lady who I saw had a little bowl of almonds at the side of her bed. These looked like healthy nibbles but in fact, they had originally been purchased as sugared almonds and the toothless lady had sucked off the sugar but could not manage the nut, which was dropped into the bowl.)

- Unlike in any other medical situation, you will be entirely dependent for diagnosis upon those very basic clinical skills taught in the first few weeks of clinical medicine. Surprisingly, if applied diligently, they work.

During the early 1980s, one of the local residential homes had an influx of old ladies who had been in Rainhill Psychiatric Hospital for, in some cases, more than fifty years. They had no psychiatric illness but had been admitted for moral degeneracy, having got pregnant underage. I suspect that they may not have been the brightest people but when the large psychiatric hospitals started to reduce their beds and close down; these ladies lacked the life-skills to enable them to manage in the real world and had to continue to live their lives in institutions. Some typhoid sufferers, whose condition could not be eradicated and who became carriers, were also similarly incarcerated in asylums for the protection of the general public.

One of my colleagues warned me to always do domiciliary visits in a timely manner. He related the story about having visited someone a few days after the request. He knocked on the door to find it answered by a young woman. He explained that he had come to see a Mrs Murphy and was shown into the house and directed to the coffin in the parlour. It was assumed that he was an acquaintance coming to pay his last respects. He carefully secreted his stethoscope out of view, said a few words, and made a hasty departure.

Paraphrenia is a psychiatric condition, predominately affecting elderly females. It has been described as the 'elderly sister of schizophrenia'. It usually manifests itself as a fixed delusion, often paranoid in nature. Such individuals can appear perfectly sane in other respects. One such lady had led a somewhat reclusive life. She believed that she was an undercover spy for the Special Branch. Her communications were through secret transmitters and receivers, hidden within her television set. She was fairly harmless but was reluctant to let anybody into her house. One wily colleague turned up one day. The door was opened on a chain. He flashed before her eyes, a form of innocent identification, announcing that he was from the Ministry of Defence, coming to give her an annual medical. He was allowed access.

Some, however, have less innocent delusions and can cause much waste of police time. One lady, living in a flat some 4 storeys high, remarked to her general practitioner that she could see a bomb-making factory in the back room of a house which she overlooked. This was at the time of the serious IRA threats. The GP didn't really take it too seriously but happened to mention it to a police inspector, with whom he was playing a round of golf. He took it more seriously. A plain clothes police officer, under the guise of being a temporary post man, made a few discrete enquiries, discovering that within the house identified, there were a bunch of young men from Northern Ireland, with strong accents. Matters were escalated to the Special Branch, who performed a dawn raid. In fact, it turned out to be quite innocent. They were students, originally from Northern Ireland, who had been brewing beer in the back kitchen. They endured the frightening experience of having their door smashed open in the early hours of the morning and being apprehended at gunpoint.

I once went to see an aging man who lived alone. He lived in a small terraced house, with the front door opening directly into the sitting room. My knock on the door was greeted with "Come in, it's open". I took two steps into the room, to be met by the sight of contentment in old age. He was sitting comfortably in his armchair, watching a pornographic video on the TV, with a can of beer, a bucket for urine and an industrial size ashtray all to hand.

One man had been awarded the George Cross during WW2 for defusing an incendiary bomb which had landed inside a gasometer. I was humbled to be allowed to see the medal, handle it and read the citation.

Anaemia is normally associated with severe weakness and tiredness. However, if it has come on exceptionally slowly, patients adapt accordingly. This is particularly the case with profound anaemia, due to either folate deficiency or pernicious anaemia from vitamin B12 deficiency. I vividly recall seeing two patients at home, with haemoglobin levels of three grams (normally, the level is over twelve grams). One lady was slowly attending to the household chores and in fact, was in the process of cooking her husband's tea when I saw her. She had the classic text-book signs. I admitted her as a matter of urgency. These chronic anaemias, due to vitamin deficiencies, do not require treatment with transfusion. They will normally respond very quickly to vitamin replacement. However, there are some dangers. They can drop dead suddenly from cardiac arrhythmias as the treatment is commenced. The body plasma in which the blood cells float is predominately water and sodium chloride, with a small amount of potassium chloride. Fluid inside the cells is predominately potassium chloride, with a small amount of sodium chloride. When profound anaemias are treated with vitamin supplementation, cells are rapidly created. The potassium to fill the cells has to come from the plasma and this can result in major shifts of potassium and consequent low blood levels, which upsets and de-stabilises the heart. This was a lesson hard learned in the 1960s and potassium supplementation was always given. That lesson has now been forgotten. I suspect it is no longer a problem, as few people are allowed to reach such low levels of haemoglobin before action is taken.

Patients who are seen at home are normally fitter than those in hospital. As a consequence, it is extremely rare for a doctor to be present in someone's house at the time of death. Since the infamous 'acts' of Dr Shipman, it is now "suspicious" if a patient's death occurs in the doctor's presence. This however has happened to me, on three occasions. On one miserable dark foggy late afternoon in December, I was asked to see an elderly man with bronchitis at home in his bungalow. I was in a rush as we had a dinner engagement that night and I was under strict orders not to be late home. I duly arrived at the patient's home, rang the doorbell and in due course, became aware of the patient struggling to walk down the hall, hampered by his breathlessness and wheezing. The door was eventually opened and we then retraced his steps, back to his bedroom. I commenced my examination and then laid him flat on the bed whilst I performed an ECG. Whilst concentrating on the dials, it flat lined. He had had a cardiac arrest. I made some attempts at cardiac resuscitation but to no avail. The soft bed did not lend itself to effective cardiac massage and whilst he had oxygen at home, it was of insufficient concentration to make any difference. He died. We were the only two in the house. Aware of my domestic responsibilities and conscious of the fact that I could no longer do anything positive, I thought of sneaking out and returning home, for him to be found in due course the following day. Fortunately, my moral compass precluded this. I alerted his general practitioner by phone. He was busy in the evening surgery and took the view that it was my problem and not his. Again, I thought of sneaking off but was ever conscious of the fact that it was not only wrong but the cover-up is always that which gets you into more serious trouble. I thought of the potential consequences. What if someone had found him, semi-undressed and alerted the police. They would then be looking for a man in a suit, who had let himself out of the house and disappeared. I would be a suspect. His phone book listed his friends, acquaintances and doubtless family, but I could gain no clue as to who was his actual next of kin. Fortunately, I went next door to find that one of the neighbours knew him well and had emergency phone contacts. The relatives lived over fifty miles away and I had to break the bad news over the phone. I tidied him up, turned down the central heating a significant number of degrees and then beetled off.

On another occasion, I was greeted by the patient's wife and introduced to the patient, who was sitting in his armchair downstairs. I made the usual introductions and suggested that he went upstairs and lay on the bed, pending my examination. After a decent interval, and after obtaining a short history from his wife, I followed him upstairs. He had died. Whether it was from the exertions of walking up the stairs, perhaps faster than normal, I know not. I felt very embarrassed, having to come downstairs and explain to his wife that a seemingly fit individual had died in my presence.

On another occasion, I arrived to find that the patient had died, probably only five minutes or so before my arrival. There was still the occasional peri-mortem gasp but no pulse.

One of the normal sights that greeted me as I drove to work each day was a short elderly man taking an enormous Irish wolfhound for its regular walk. I happened to meet him again in the role of patient's husband on a domiciliary visit. His wife was bedbound in a bedroom downstairs and her budgies were flying around the room. The Irish wolfhound greeted me with some suspicion and whilst I was undertaking the examination, sat 'on guard'. Whilst I was listening to her chest with the stethoscope, out of the corner of my eye, I spotted the dog opening and shutting his mouth rapidly. I realised that he had eaten one of the budgies. I pointed this out, to be informed that this was fairly common. The man told me that, whether true or not, budgerigar was Aboriginal for 'good to eat'.

Vary rarely was the general practitioner in actual attendance. On one occasion, I attended a patient whose elderly general practitioner had wished to be present. When I arrived, I found that the old doctor had tripped over the patient's cat and had sustained a head injury and fractured his arm. The patient had already called an ambulance. I visited another man, who lived in a house on a street with a residential care home for delinquent teenagers. As I drew up in the car, a group of youths were hurling significant sized stones at his windows. Rather than risk their assault being redirected to my car, I very politely asked them to desist, at least whilst I was in performing an examination. They reluctantly complied. The patient was completely undaunted by this action. It had been problematic a few years before but he had solved the problem by installing bulletproof glass throughout the house (his son was a glazier, who was able to source the glass locally, at cost price).

Use of oxygen at home is now fairly commonplace. This was not the case thirty years ago, as it was fraught with practical difficulties. The small cylinders of oxygen for domestic use had to be replaced frequently and could be dangerous in the presence of a naked flame. For many years, oxygen concentrators which merely concentrate the oxygen in the air have been used to provide a marginally higher dose to be inhaled through a mask. District nurses can get quite anxious about patients with oxygen concentrators being used in houses with open fires, gas fires and even gas hobs in the kitchen. This is quite unnecessary. One patient, who I saw at home, had been threatened by a rather bossy district nurse, that she would take his oxygen away unless he converted his fire. I was able to demonstrate that this was unnecessary by lighting a cigarette lighter next to the oxygen discharge pipe to show that it merely made the flame glow a little stronger. There was no danger of explosion.

When I started doing domiciliary visits in the early 1980s, it was common practice to be offered an alcoholic drink. I suspect this practice said more about the patient's general practitioner than anything else. One wag once pointed out that an alcoholic is someone who drinks more than his doctor.

During the great freeze of January 1983, when temperatures barely rose above 0°C for a week or more, I struggled to visit an old lady in her home. Her upstairs water tank had burst, cascading water throughout the house. She was sitting in the living room, under an umbrella, to protect herself from the dripping water. The water main had fortunately been turned off. The electrics, however, were unaffected, simply because she had no electricity. She had rented the house for over 50 years and had resisted the landlord's offer to install electricity. Her lighting was still by old fashioned gas lights.

One of the great unsolved murder mysteries of all time is the murder of Julia Wallace, at her home in Richmond Park, Liverpool, in January 1931. In short, Julia Wallace had been bludgeoned to death. Her husband was initially arrested and found guilty but acquitted on appeal. His alibi was that he had been sent on a wild goose chase, to a fictitious address at the other end of the city. The murder occurred at 29 Wolverton Street which, for years afterwards, would attract sightseers. I went to see an elderly brother and sister, who resided in Wolverton Street, across the road from the murder scene. This elderly pair had been children at the time, and were still living in the same house. They were able to give me a first-hand account of the events as they had seen them unfold.

I obtained insight into the consequences of lifetime choices, when I visited an elderly couple living in severe poverty, in a small council flat. They were cultured individuals. Both of them had university degrees but had largely been shunned by their peers. They had become Communists whilst at university in the 1930s and had gone to Spain to fight with the International Brigades against Franco, during the civil war. He had taken up arms, whilst she was a camp follower, who had assisted, as-and-when with the various back room tasks of administration and occasional nursing. To be involved in warfare as a combatant, in any circumstances, can be a grim affair. However, civil wars are much more vicious, in that grudges can mean that the normal rules of war under the Geneva Convention are largely ignored. The medical services for the injured are less organised and can even be very primitive. Although she had no formal nursing background, her observation was that badly contaminated wounds had the best chance of survival if they were full of maggots on arrival at field dressing stations. This lesson had been learned in the American civil war but had been largely forgotten thereafter. It was once again forgotten after the Spanish civil war, but maggot therapy has now been standard for some years, to treat deep grade 4 pressure sores. Maggots will not eat live tissue but they will eradicate dead and contaminated flesh, with their vigorous appetites. This couple had a deep-seated belief in the fairness of Communism. They had held on to that belief through thick and thin, despite the effect it had on their careers. No one would employ them. Police and the security services hassled them repeatedly, yet they still remained true to their faith with the expectation that within their lifetime, capitalism would be defeated and communism hold sway. When I saw them, it was the time of the collapse of the Berlin wall, when the Soviet Union was jettisoning Communist ideals. They both became deeply depressed, having realised their lifetime sacrifice had been to no avail.

Some houses can be extremely spooky. One man I saw lived in a house where every room had a big colourful picture of the all-seeing eye, embellished with the slogan in large letters 'Thy God Seeth Everything'. Another house I visited was a big dark end-of-terrace. The windows received little sun and that which it did receive naturally was obscured by overgrown bushes. The occupant was an old lady of a reclusive nature, whose only companion was the ghost of her dead nephew. Much of our conversation involved him as a third party.

On two occasions, I have visited museum pieces. On both occasions, the occupants were single individuals who had been widowed young. One elderly man had lost his young wife during child birth. The baby had also died. Nothing in that house had changed from her death, in 1923. It had become a shrine to her memory. He still cooked on the range, which surrounded the fire, in the back living room. There was no internal running water apart from one cold tap in the "scullery" and the toilet was outside. Her tombstone had been photographed and the photo hung in the parlour. It had the poignant inscription 'Twenty years a maiden/one year a wife/one hour a mother, and then I lost my life'. He had clearly not gotten over the upset.

Another patient had lost her young husband in the final days of WW1. Once again, her home had become a shrine to his memory, though some of her domestic appliances had been updated. I was asked to see her because she was hallucinating. After some sixty years in his grave, her husband was now visiting her on a nightly basis and sitting with her in the evenings. She gained great comfort from his presence and eagerly awaited her demise, such that they would be reunited. Professional opinion was evenly split as to the moral right and wisdom to deprive her of this by prescribing potent antipsychotic drugs. Those who knew her well, claimed that they had never seen her happier. I advised leaving matters as they were. I was informed that she remained happy and died peacefully in her bed, some months later.

One odd condition, which geriatricians regularly see is the Senile Squalor Syndrome. The Senile Squalor syndrome, sometimes called Diogenes syndrome, is an unusual condition seen mostly, but not exclusively, in elderly people. Over the age of 60, approximately 1 person per 2000 is affected per year. The condition is not a disease as such and is not a psychiatric illness, as these people show no evidence of psychiatric disease. It appears to be a positive reaction against the usual standards of personal and environmental hygiene and may represent the end stage of a lifelong personality disorder. The main features are as follows:

- Gross self-neglect.

- Social isolation.

- Extreme squalor.

- Indifference to their surroundings.

- Often an extremely offensive odour in and around the house.

- Rubbish hoarding and reluctance to tidy or to throw anything out.

In their younger days, these people were usually of normal to high intelligence, previously socially competent and usually held down responsible jobs. Often there is past evidence of an independent streak, with them becoming gradually more reclusive, stubborn and quarrelsome as the years progress. They mostly live alone, with a preponderance of females to males.

The deterioration in their personality and social functioning is often gradual but occasionally follows a specific life-changing event, such as the death of a spouse, or change in domestic relationships. It is not related to poverty, and mobility outside the home is usually well preserved for many years. They are very reluctant to allow people into their homes and offers of help are almost always refused. They may be well known to social services and environmental health departments. It is not unusual for the utility supplies to have been discontinued for either safety reasons or non-payment of bills.

This syndrome has a wide spectrum, ranging from relatively mild but still significant and abnormal self-neglect, through to extreme examples, which may make newspaper headlines

I have seen some ten cases as part of my clinical practice and a further thirty to forty across the country, for various criminal and civilian legal reasons. My first case in routine practice involved visiting a large double fronted Victorian house, which had fallen into disrepair. It was partially boarded up and appeared, to the casual observer, to be unoccupied. The whole two storeys of one of the front walls, to the right of the front door, had collapsed. The roof was propped up with some scaffolding and a large tarpaulin sheet kept out the elements. In fact, it was occupied by an elderly lady and her daughter. The daughter had a history of schizophrenia but was functional and taking no medication. The old lady was bedbound and had developed a large pressure sore. The heroines in this piece were the team of district nurses, who had been visiting on a daily basis to provide some home treatment. Three dogs were present. When anyone approached the front door, one small dog – the watchdog – would emerge from behind the tarpaulin and bark, standing on the front door porch roof. That would alert the guard dogs, one aggressive Alsatian and an enormous English mastiff. They would join him on the porch and bark at anyone at the door. The mastiff would drool saliva on the heads of those outside. Despite the attentions of the district nurses, matters were worsening and they were concerned about her health and wellbeing, given that the house was piled high with hoarded rubbish. There were small narrow passages wending their way throughout piles of bales of hoarded newspapers, magazines and rubbish. The old lady in her double bed was in the front bedroom, which was basically only protected from the elements by the tarpaulin. The source of heat was an ancient electric fire, positioned on the floor and dangerously close to the bed clothes and the newspaper piles. Scorch marks to some of the newspapers and the counterpane bore witness to the obvious dangers. I was asked to visit and ran the gauntlet of the dogs before proceeding upstairs. Turning back the bedsheets revealed an enormous necrotic grade 4 pressure sore. This was deep, highly offensive and had eroded through her buttocks and into her pelvic bones. The dogs pushed me aside and started to lick it. She also shared her bed with half of a cow's skeleton; the bones were clearly gnawing bones for the dogs. The whole circumstance was completely appalling. I overruled her wishes and insisted on hospitalisation. As I learned later, with more experience, this was probably the worst thing that I could have done. I used the blunt instrument of the Section 47 Act, (only very recently repealed) the details of which were as follows:

Section 47 of the 1948 National Assistance Act

Section 47 of the 1948 National Assistance Act gave the Medical Officer of Health the power to apply to a Magistrate for the compulsory removal of persons who:

i) Are suffering from grave chronic disease or being aged, infirm or physically incapacitated, are living in insanitary conditions.

ii) Are unable to devote to themselves and are not receiving from other persons, proper care and attention.

It required 7 days' notice to authorise a person's detention in a suitable hospital or other place, for a period not exceeding 3 months. During the 7 days' period of notice, matters could and in one widely publicised case, did deteriorate dramatically, which led to the Act being amended as below.

National Assistance (Amendment) Act of 1951

This allowed compulsory removal to be immediate, provided that the opinion of the Medical Officer of Health was supported by that of another Registered Medical Practitioner. It is considered to be best practice for a geriatrician to be in that supporting role.

The period of detention was limited to 3 weeks. This Act, although used about 250 times per annum in the UK during the 1980's, was little known about outside very specialised medical circles. I have assessed about 10 patients in the role of 'another Registered Medical Practitioner' but only twice, in nearly 30 years as a Consultant, have I found all the elements required to be present. Compulsory removal is associated with a high mortality rate, and as such, may not be in the person's best interest, and should not be done without overwhelming reason. Immediately following hospitalisation, she basically 'gave up' and died.

Brucellosis is an infectious bacterial disease, normally acquired from infected animals and particularly

146

from their milk. The milk of cows, sheep and goats and soft cheeses made therefrom are the usual sources. It is exceptionally rare in the UK and has almost entirely been eradicated by pasteurisation of milk and good farm practices. It is characterised by fever, which in chronic form can be relapsing. On one occasion, I was asked to see an elderly Greek man, who spoke no English. I visited him in the home of his daughter-in-law on a council estate. She was English and widowed. By courtesy of the regular Easy Jet flights between Liverpool and Athens, she was able to return frequently to visit her extended family. Her father-in-law Demetrius lived on and ran a small farm outside Athens. He had been taken ill some weeks before and hospitalised in Athens. As far as she was aware, he had received a course of treatment and been discharged home. She had brought him back to her house for a period of convalescence. When I saw him, he was ensconced in the box-room, surrounded by religious icons and fervently praying. She had kept a temperature chart, which showed a relapsing fever, coming and going over a period of some days. There were no localising clinical signs and in particular, his chest was clear. There was no obvious cause. She had brought with her copies of his hospital records but these were all in the Greek alphabet. My Greek at the best of times is poor and this defeated me. I could identify from the results in the discharge notes that he had been tested for brucellosis but could not work out whether or not that was the actual diagnosis. I did however suspect that brucellosis might be the diagnosis here. I phoned up the Department of Infectious Diseases, who were extremely sceptical, rightly pointing out that sparrows are more common than canaries in Liverpool gardens. I needed more ammunition. With the daughter-in-law's permission, I borrowed the records and hared back to the hospital. I knew of a trainee public health doctor who was Greek in origin. After a few phone calls and faxing of the appropriate pages, it turned out that the man had been admitted to hospital in Athens and diagnosed as having brucellosis. The antibiotics he had been given were not the most effective and he had probably taken them for too short a course. Armed with that information, I was able to re-contact the Infectious Disease department and arrange his admission. He did have brucellosis and he made a full recovery.

Chronic leg ulcers occupy a great deal of district nursing time. They need frequent dressings and a high degree of vigilance to make sure that infection does not set in within the surrounding tissues. On a number of occasions, I have been asked to see such patients where the district nurses have become extremely perturbed because the patient is letting their dogs and cats lick the ulcers clean. My experience is that this rarely causes problems and in fact, the literature suggests that this is more beneficial, than harmful.

A man in his late 70s was referred to my outpatient clinic with the sudden onset of confusion. He was given an appointment to come to the hospital, some ten days later. In the meantime, his wife had phoned up, claiming he was too unwell to attend. My response, after consultation with his GP, was to do a home visit. The story was as follows: They had gone on holiday to Crete. He had been the usual 'man in charge' dealing with the tickets and passports and negotiating the check-in desk, etc., with ease. He had been swimming in the sea and generally behaving like an exceptionally fit man for his age. Some mid-way through their fortnight holiday, he had started to show a degree of disinterest in matters and by the end of the holiday, he was too confused to take charge of the travel arrangements. The usual cause of sudden onset confusion is either a delirium from infection or small strokes, which can lead to rapid onset of a vascular dementia. There were no signs of infection on examination and he had minimal, if any, vascular risk factors. He warranted further investigation and I arranged his admission. His only significant previous medical history was that his cataracts had been operated upon, some months before.

Within days of his admission, he significantly deteriorated from a neurological perspective. One of the ward sisters, whose friend had died from variant CJD, noted some obscure twitching. On more detailed observation, this was clearly myoclonus. Myoclonus is the twitching of individual muscles, rather than muscle fibres of a more generalised nature. It can be a hallmark of CJD. My suspicions were aroused. Many people had heard of the variant form of CJD, known as mad cow disease, which peaked during the 1990s, as a result of people eating the meat from infected cattle. There is however an older form, the sporadic non-variant form of CJD, which has a more rapid onset. This is what I suspected. I arranged for him to be seen by a neurologist but in the two days before he was seen, he continued to deteriorate. I was fairly confident about my diagnosis and was aware that the instruments used to operate upon his cataracts may have been contaminated. I did not suspect the cataract operation was the cause of his CJD, but of more concern to me was that those instruments may be still in use and could potentially infect other patients, if I were right. Pending diagnostic confirmation, I suggested that the instruments, which had been used upon him, should be temporarily put out of circulation (such instruments can be identified quite easily).

That seemed a straightforward sensible request to me. It was eventually done, but only after lots of hand wringing, as to whether patients who may have been operated upon subsequently, ought to be informed even though nothing had been proven. In any event, he deteriorated rapidly and died. The only way to confirm the diagnosis was by post mortem examination. However, the infectious agent, a prion, is indestructible and there was great reluctance to undergo post mortem, for fear of contaminating people, instruments and indeed, the post mortem suite. Eventually, and using particularly strenuous precautions, a limited post mortem was done, and the brain removed. The centre for CJD research was in Edinburgh. Of course, Scotland has completely different legal rules and there was a lot of complex red-tape to deal with before an English Coroner would allow body parts to go 'abroad'. Eventually, the diagnosis of sporadic CJD was confirmed. A handful of patients, who had had their eyes operated on with the potentially contaminated instruments, were informed of the possible, but low risk, of contamination. There was and is no treatment. It struck me as being a little pointless to worry people about the possibility of acquiring something for which nothing could be done. To have said nothing might have been kinder – this would not have been a cover-up because no-one had done anything wrong. As the instruments were exclusively used for cataract surgery and most people with cataracts are effectively retired, the chances of them actually getting CJD, within their likely life expectancy, would be vanishingly small. CJD probably has an incubation period of twenty to thirty years.

CHAPTER EIGHT

The Natural World

Domiciliary visiting provides a fascinating insight into the relationship of people with animals. I once read some research from the University of Bristol which concluded that cat owners were cleverer than dog owners. University graduates were significantly more likely than the general population to own a cat, whereas dog ownership was generally associated with more modest educational achievement. Today's dogs are apparently descended from a pack of wolves, tamed some sixteen thousand years ago, on the shores of the Yangzi River in China. The domestication of the dog seemed to coincide with the transformation of the population in that part of the world from hunter gatherers to farmers. Dogs apparently enjoy travelling at speed, with their heads out of car windows, because it is the thrilling equivalent of a hunting charge, spearheaded by the leader of the pack, who is the car driver. Their ultra-sensitive noses are exposed to a heady mixture of unfamiliar but fascinating roadside smells. I once came across the case of a police drug-sniffer dog, which had to be put down, after it developed a rather rare nasal cancer. Whether that cancer had an occupational cause, I know not. A magistrate once told me of a dog owner who lost his driving licence, after he was caught walking the animal, whilst he was driving down the street, holding the lead through the window. There was also the case of a 42-year-old grandmother, caught on camera, having sex with the family Rottweiler pet. She had taken 'selfie' photographs and although they did not show her face, she was readily identified by some unique tattoos. A police dog, released in Dorset to chase some armed robbers, was reported in the press as having gone off message and killed a sheep and savaged two others, before being recalled. A vet told me about operating on a dog, expecting to find a tumour in the golden retriever but found, to his surprise, enough clothes to fill a small washing line. The clothes were assorted gloves, a mitten, a stocking and a dozen socks. It had apparently been eating the assorted garments for years and they were removed one-by-one, like a conjuring trick. One of my friends had a Labrador, which had eaten a pair of baby's knitted tights. This became apparent whilst the dog was squatting and straining at stool. One leg of the faeces filled tight emerged, to the distance of one foot but would not detach. The dog kept turning to look, with a sad expression. The problem was solved quite quickly by putting one foot on the tip of the leg and encouraging the dog to run off, by gently tapping its rear end with his other foot. The gusset and the other leg of the tights emerged as the dog bounded freely ahead. I am told that the other children refused to allow the parents to use those tights again, even after they had been washed!

Our neighbour's dog died after eating a bag of sultanas. This is apparently a common problem, with dogs being very susceptible to becoming sick after eating grapes, raisins or sultanas. The toxins from the fruit cause renal failure, which is basically untreatable. They are also very sensitive to theobromine, which is a stimulant found in chocolate. This affects the central nervous system as well as the heart muscle and can easily kill a dog. Special dog chocolate is of course available. Normally, one reads in the paper about dog owners drowning in an attempt to save their pet. One dog, who was saved from a swollen river, repaid his rescuer by savaging its arm.

Police in Lincolnshire received a phone call at eight o'clock in the morning, from a concerned member of the public who had been parked in a layby, next to a busy road and adjacent to some woodland. A white van had arrived and two men jumped out. They opened the rear doors of the van and struggled to remove a heavy object, wrapped in a roll of carpet. Armed with a shovel each, they carried their burden into the woods, remerging an hour later. Police attended the scene and followed the trail of heavy footprints, some hundred yards, to a clearing. There was evidence of fresh digging and a muddy trail led back to the layby but the van had gone. The decision as to what to do next was escalated. Eventually, an Inspector sent the SOCO Team. Other police cordoned off the scene and a mobile incident room took over the layby. By now, some ten members of staff were involved. Layer by layer, soil was removed, with the operation being videoed for evidential purposes. Some three feet down, a roll of carpet became exposed. It was wrapped around something 'warmish' and soft. Photographs were taken and the carpet peeled back, to reveal a body of a recently dead Alsatian dog. This was disinterred. After a final check below to make sure that nothing extra had been buried below the dog, the hole was filled in and the dog's body taken for incineration.

'Mice killed the cats', read the newspaper headline. Nearly one hundred cats at a Canadian animal shelter, died in a fire, which was probably caused by mice chewing through electrical wires in the ceiling of the building. Fire also destroyed a family home when kittens turned on the gas by walking across a touch sensitive hob. A pet rat once caused a fire when it grabbed a smouldering cigarette butt from the owner's ashtray and hid it in the hay inside its open cage. During the night, the cigarette continued to burn and eventually set the cage and the room alight.

One cat in ten is now believed to suffer from dementia, as the feline population ages. Signs of the disease include getting disorientated, with cats being trapped in corners or failing to find the litter tray. Crying at night and aggressive behaviour are recognised features, together with attention seeking activities, altered sleeping patterns and disinterest in food, together with aimless wandering and decreased grooming. One cat owner was awoken from sleep, by police attending a 999 call. They insisted that 999 had been dialled from his house, yet he was asleep. The culprit was apparently his cat, who was asleep next to the phone, which was off the hook. It was concluded that it was the cat who had dialled 999 with its paw, whilst sleeping. An American Geriatrician, Dr David Dosa, wrote an article in the New England Journal of Medicine, back in 2007, about a cat called Oscar, which was resident within a nursing home, in Rhode Island. The cat had been adopted as a kitten but was generally antisocial and rarely spent significant time with residents. However, it had the uncanny knack of identifying those with just hours to live. It could identify the imminent death and would stretch itself out on the resident's bed. If doors were closed, it would scratch and mew, until admitted. Apparently, nurses once placed the cat on the bed of a patient they thought close to death. Oscar charged out and went to sit beside someone else. The cat's judgement was better than that of the nurses, as the second patient died that evening, whilst the first lived for two more days. Casper, a twelve-year-old cat from Plymouth, made the headlines when it was revealed that he regularly caught the same bus from outside its home. He caught the number 3 bus, at 10.00 am each morning, and rode on the back seat for the entire eleven mile round-trip journey. The drivers had been instructed to ensure that the cat got off at the right stop. Sadly, after doing this for some four years, Caspar was run over whilst racing for the bus. There was talk that his story would be made into a children's book. One ginger 'tom' went missing from the south coast and despite the owners putting up posters and handing out leaflets, there was no sign. Some four days later, they received a phone call. The cat had taken a ship to Bilbao in Northern Spain.

Cat flaps are not without their problems. Our eldest daughter was awoken at 03.00 am on Christmas morning by a cat fight in her front hall. Two aggressive cats had followed their pussy indoors and were causing havoc. The problem was solved by re-jigging the cat flap with some magnetic device that only allowed their cat to open it. However, she also collected various items of cutlery and regularly used to get attached to the radiator. For a while, we had an unneutered ginger 'tom' that enjoyed nocturnal meanderings. His territory overlapped with that of a larger ginger 'tom', also living in the neighbourhood. Late one night, as we were going to sleep, we heard the mewing of ours and another cat outside our front door. I went downstairs to investigate, to find our cat cowering in the corner, being threatened by its larger rival. I went to shew him away, armed with a yard brush and our cat hared off, but the neighbour's cat ran up the brush and I was lucky not to have my eyes scratched out. Sometime later, our cat received a severe eye injury from a scratch in a cat fight, but refused attention. He basically ran off, only to return some days later, with its eyeball full of pus. We took it to the vet and followed their advice. In one operation, the cat had its eyeball removed and it was also castrated. It wore a large collar to protect its eye from being scratched and clearly could not lie or sit comfortably for a few days. It did however eventually recover, only to succumb some years later from a wasting condition, which may have been feline leukaemia virus or cat HIV. In his younger days and presumably due to testosterone fuelled promiscuity, our cat was prone to fleas. He could remove all flea collars within days and needed periodic spraying with a proprietary flea killer. This he hated. He developed an uncanny sense as to when it was due to be treated and would disappear. Not to be thwarted and armed with the can, I chased him around the house and eventually out into the garden, where I managed to catch his tail in a rugby tackle. I sprayed liberally. Both cat and I were enveloped in the spray, the children were not amused at the sight they beheld, the cat being firmly gripped by tail, whilst I was lying on the floor, spraying in a maniacal manner. The cat was foaming at the mouth, I was drooling and my vision had gone off. I realised what had happened. The flea spray was an organophosphate, which was basically nerve gas. {Nerve gases are chemical warfare agents with the same action as organophosphate insecticides. They are both potent inhibitors of acetylcholinesterase. Inhibition of this leads to an accumulation of acetylcholine in the central and peripheral nervous system. Excess acetylcholine produces the predictable cholinergic syndrome consisting of copious respiratory and oral secretions, diarrhoea and vomiting, sweating, altered mental status, autonomic instability, and generalized weakness that can progress to paralysis and respiratory arrest.} At the time, these insecticides were in regular use and particularly so for sheep dipping. Many farmers developed significant problems of a neurological nature after repeated exposure, but I seem to have gotten away with that one.

Charles Darwin was fascinated with barnacles and recorded the significant problems with their sex life. The male barnacle rooted to the spot, had to constantly wave his penis, erected at the cost of lots of hydraulic energy, to reach out and tap its neighbours, in the hope that at least one might be female. The organ of one species was particularly wonderfully developed, being between eight and nine times the entire length of the animal. Pedigree animals are sometimes reluctant to engage in sex, rather defeating the purpose of keeping them for stud. One enterprising vet had an international reputation for stimulating the sex drive of pedigree stallions. The techniques included placing blankets soaked in mare's urine on their backs and even introducing reluctant thoroughbreds to a harem of cart horses, in the hope that they may be stimulated by 'rough trade'. Pedigree Bull dogs tend to mate naturally, without difficulty. However, they can't be left alone. The best advice is for the owner of the bitch to hold its head to ensure that it does not turn around and bite the face of the dog. Dogs so bitten in their sensitive jowls during intercourse tend not to go back for more and they can be put off mating for life. A pedigree bull, reluctant to perform, was facing slaughter but was saved by using Viagra. {If you put Viagra drops in both eyes it makes you look "dead hard". Don't get the Viagra virus on an old computer – it'll turn your 3.5-inch floppy into hard drive. Thieves who stole a lorry-load of Viagra were hardened criminals, who got long, stiff sentences}.

Periodically, mummified cats are found walled up in old houses being renovated. Some four hundred years ago, it was common practice to put cats behind the walls to ward off witches and act as some kind of good luck charm. The Doberman was created in the 1860s by a German tax collector, to protect him against obvious occupational hazards. I have it on good authority that brown eggs are laid by hens with red or brown earlobes and that white eggs are laid by hens with white earlobes.

A goldfish was reported in the press as surviving for thirteen hours on the floor after leaping from its bowl. Apparently, fish can survive quite a long while out of water, as long as their gills remain moist. Bats are protected species and tend to fly through railway tunnels and some colonies also roost there during the day. Chiltern railways came up with a solution by installing lights in one such tunnel, which would come on as a train approached. Bats apparently do not like bright lights and when a train approached, the lights would come on and they would leave the area, avoiding being hit and killed. Bat colonies in churches regularly cause problems. Bat droppings can ruin ancient brasses. Country graveyards can attract badgers, who like nothing better than digging up human bones. Anyone who has had moles in their garden will know the damage which they can cause. There are some practical ways to keep the moles at bay:

- A mole barrier can be created by digging a trench, three feet deep and twelve inches wide, around the area you wish to protect. It ought to be filled with gravel and then covered up.

- If moles are already present, a pit trap can be created. Basically, dig into the mole tunnel and place a very large jar deep in the ground, with the rim level with the bottom of the tunnel. Cover the tunnel with material to keep the light out and check the trap regularly.

- A garden hose inserted into the mole tunnel and turned on, will cause it to flood and the moles to leave.

- Pouring castor oil into a mole's tunnel might give it an upset stomach and discourage it from staying.

- Mouse traps also work.

The rise in mole numbers coincided with the EU ban on the use of strychnine, in 2006. No other bait poison can be legally used to control moles. The remaining chemical option is aluminium phosphide gas, which being heavier than air, can permeate tunnels, killing not only moles but anything else it encounters. There has been a rise in suicides from use of this gas, which I am told renders the body extremely toxic, making post mortem examination dangerous. The mole is still toasted by Jacobites, as the 'little gentleman in black velvet'. This is thought to be because a mole hill brought down William III when he was riding at Hampton Court. The King broke his collar bone and three weeks later was dead.

Bees in the wrong place can cause chaos. Two hives of bees were smuggled onto a plane for a flight across

Russia and escaped in mid-air, swarming around the cabin. This led to an emergency landing and a hasty evacuation of the plane. Bees are regularly transported around the USA to assist with the pollination of field crops. One trailer, carrying seven thousand bee hives with an estimated seventeen million bees, crashed on a highway. Rescue crews had to use fire hoses to douse the angry swarms, which were interfering with the rescue operation. At one point, honey bees were being trained to sniff out explosives for use at airports. Bees were trained to extend their proboscis when smelling a particular explosive and could be placed into a sniffer box. A slug brought cars to a standstill when it crawled into a set of traffic lights and short circuited the electrics.

The urban fox population is thought to number in excess of thirty-three thousand, compared to a quarter of a million living in the countryside. They were first noted in towns and cities in the 1940s, but numbers have risen since. In some big cities, there are estimated to be up to thirty foxes per square mile. Their diet is mostly made up of rats, mice, pigeons, rabbits, worms and insects, with probably up to a third obtained by scavenging from household rubbish. They hunt alone but live in family groups, with their dens commonly being under garden sheds or decking. The life expectancy of an urban fox is less than two years, mainly because disease spreads more quickly. Urban foxes are known to kill domestic cats and periodically, foxes are reported to break into houses and savage children. These tend to be mature cubs, which are starting to explore. Some years ago, a suburb of a Kentish town was plagued with attacks of apparent sabotage on cars. During an eight month period, some ten vehicles had their brake pipes cut. The police investigation involved forensically examining the vehicles and CCTV footage was studied, to try and identify the culprit. The cuts and marks left on the vehicle components were eventually identified as being made by an animal, probably a fox. The local foxes had apparently developed a taste for brake fluid.

Rudolph the red nose reindeer was almost certainly female. Male reindeer grow antlers for the mating season in the autumn but they are usually cast off before Christmas. By contrast, female reindeer grow their antlers in time for winter, in order to compete with other females over holes they dig in the snow to reach the lichens and to provide food for their offspring.

Pet animals often provide excuses for avoiding parking fines. In one case, the traffic warden accepted that the parrot, loose inside a vehicle, had knocked the resident's parking permit off the dashboard and cancelled the ticket. A driver who parked outside a vet, in order to take in a sick python, claimed that he should not have been expected to carry the poorly creature through the streets. That appeal was rejected.

A town in New Zealand was forced to cancel a historic rabbit throwing competition after complaints from animal rights groups. Before the annual pig hunt, children in the small town had traditionally competed to see how far they could throw a dead rabbit. The RSPCA had protested that the contest sent the wrong message to children, in that dead animals could legitimately be used as a form of entertainment. Surrey police were alerted by a 999 call to the fact of a giant turquoise flying rabbit, which had drifted passed someone's house, with a passenger on its back. It was in fact a partially deflated helium balloon in the shape of a rabbit. This was discovered after it crashed into a bridge. There was no one with it. A giant white rabbit, some two feet long and twenty pounds in weight, was found roaming the streets of Canterbury, shortly after midnight. It was reported in the local press that the rabbit gave two police officers the run-around for over twenty minutes, before they enlisted the help of night clubbers, who assisted in its apprehension. An Australian zoo had to be evacuated after an ape short-circuited the electric fence, by jamming a stick into the wire. It then piled up debris to climb a wall and then sat upon the fence, before changing its mind and returning to its enclosure. Australia has thousands of camels in the remote outback. They were first introduced into Australia in the 1840s to help explorers travel and the current ones are the descendants of those set free. The population has been growing and requires periodic culling, because of the havoc they wreak. They are estimated to be some million and they compete with sheep and cattle for food and invade remote settlements in search of water.

The turning out of pigs to forage for acorns in the autumn has been a feature of woodland life for centuries. This is known as the pannage, however, apart from providing free nutrients for the pigs, there may be another reason. Acorns are toxic to horses and it was essential to keep down the numbers, which they might be tempted to eat. Since the rail industry started, carriages have been infested with insects. It is estimated that the average railway carriage, even now, is home to as many as a thousand cockroaches, two hundred bed bugs and two hundred fleas. The cockroaches tend to hide behind the lighting and ceiling panels, whilst the bed bugs and fleas live in the seating fabric. Years of spraying insecticide has failed to reduce their numbers. Periodically, carriages are taken out of service and heated to some 60°C, in order to kill the bugs and their eggs. In this way, the whole carriage is treated, whereas the spray leaves untreated pockets. Whilst cockroaches have a terrible reputation and are often symbols of dirt and disease, they do not actually carry disease themselves. There are thousands of species, with 99% living outdoors. They are said to be one of the most successful creatures on earth. They are able to resist around fifteen times the level of radiation that a human being can stand and they can live on just one meal a month. The cockroach is said to be able to live up to a month after decapitation, before it ends up starving to death. The severed head can also live a number of hours.

It is believed that girls are born with a natural fear of spiders. Researchers found that female babies, less than a year old, already associate spiders with fear, unlike boys, who are unconcerned. The findings, published in the New Scientist, suggest that girls may be genetically predisposed to fearing potentially deadly animals, as they presented a special danger to prehistoric women, whose children could have died without them. Traditionally, conkers placed in rooms discourages the autumnal ingress of spiders. The use of insects as weapons of war has been described in the book Six Legged Soldiers, by Jeffrey Lockwood. Probably, sometime in ancient history, someone threw a bees' nest into an enemy's fortifications; whilst the defenders were distracted, the besiegers could move in. Mongol troops used a siege engine to hurl corpses of plague victims over walls, thereby delivering a cargo of plague carrying fleas, which eagerly sought living hosts. During the WW2, the Japanese developed a research facility, whereby prisoners were deliberately infected with plague, in order to provide a source for the disease, which they could use to contaminate fleas. The fleas were harvested and packed into pottery bomb cases, which, when dropped, shattered and released their lethal cargo. The general in charge avoided prosecution after the war and allegedly went to America to advise the US military on their own insect war programme. It is alleged that British forces, operating in North America, before independence, deliberately exposed native Indians to smallpox, through infected blankets.

The puffer fish, which can blow itself up to two or three times its size to make it less vulnerable to predators, contains tetrodotoxin, which is a powerful neurotoxin, deadly to human beings and over a thousand times more poisonous than cyanide. There is said to be enough toxin in one puffer fish to kill thirty adults and there is no known antidote. Symptoms can include dizziness, exhaustion, headache, nausea and eventually asphyxiation and death can occur within minutes. Despite this, the meat is considered a delicacy in Japan and can only be prepared and cooked by trained chefs, who must remove the toxic ovaries, liver and skin. The meat is called fugu and the training of the chef takes place over a three year apprenticeship. There is an exam, with a failure rate of 60%. Eating such meals must be the culinary equivalent of Russian roulette. Much more commonly seen is scombroid poisoning. The darker flesh in some fish, for example, salmon, mackerel and tuna, is composed of protein, which has a high percentage of the amino acid histidine. If this decomposes, it is converted to histamine (as anyone with allergies well knows, histamine is the means by which the manifestations of the allergy are produced in the human body). I first came across this whilst on holiday in Venice. A member of our party had been suddenly taken ill after a meal of grilled fish. To all intents and purpose, she was thought to have had a heart attack. She developed nausea, facial flushing, vomiting, intense epigastric/chest pain and urticaria within a few minutes and was rushed to hospital in a water ambulance. She settled rapidly within twelve hours and re-joined the group for continuation of the holiday. I learnt that this is a particular problem in Venice due to the fishing techniques. Fishermen spread out their lines, baited with hooks, in the lagoon. They are harvested once daily. The lagoon waters are warm and the fish, when retrieved, may have been dead in the water, on the hook, for up to twenty-four hours. It is the bacterial decomposition of the dark meat, which converts the histidine into histamine. The fish looks fresh, smells fresh and there is no way of anticipating the contamination. It is probably best to remove the dark meat, rather than eat it.

Paralytic shellfish poisoning tends to be seasonal, occurring between June and October, if mussels, clams, oysters and scallops ingest a poisonous red algae which produces a neurotoxin that is not destroyed by cooking. The first symptoms appear within thirty minutes after ingestion and consist of numbness around the mouth, nausea, vomiting and abdominal cramps. Muscle weakness follows, with paralysis of the limbs. Respiratory paralysis can cause death. Oysters were allegedly introduced by the Romans, who enjoyed them as a delicacy. The ancient Britons previously saw shellfish as subsistence food, handy in times of need but not actively sought when fish or meat was to be had. Oysters lost their status as a delicacy after the Romans left but their popularity was gradually regained, reaching the peak of popularity during the Victorian period. Overfishing reduced the natural oyster beds. One owner of a profitable oyster bed off the Sussex coast noted that the local council had rerouted the sewers. In search of the nutrients therein, he relocated his oyster beds, to take advantage of the effluent. Disaster struck at a banquet in 1902, when several of the diners died, following typhoid. That led to a temporary collapse in the shellfish industry. Under modern hygiene regulations, all oysters are now cleaned, before being purified by ultraviolet treatment. However, intermittent poisoning can still occur, with Noro virus. It is said 'a noise annoys an oyster but a noisy noise annoys an oyster more'.

Poisoning has a long history in the political world and so alarmed the public in medieval Britain that in 1531, Henry VII passed the Poisoning Act, decreeing that all convicted poisoners should be boiled alive. Traditionally a weapon of women, arsenic was a popular way of murdering people, until recently, partly because of its availability and the difficulty of detecting it in the human body. It was sometimes referred to as "inheritance powder". In April 1889, Florence Maybrick bought flypaper containing arsenic from a local chemist's shop and later soaked it in a bowl of water. James Maybrick was taken ill on 27 April 1889 and died at his home in Battle crease House Aigburth on 11 May 1889. Florence Maybrick was charged with his murder and stood trial at St George's Hall, Liverpool. At her trial, she claimed that this method allowed her to extract the arsenic for cosmetic use. She was convicted and sentenced to death. After a public outcry, Henry Matthews, the Home Secretary, and Lord Chancellor Halsbury concluded "that the evidence clearly establishes that Mrs Maybrick administered poison to her husband with intent to murder; but that there is ground for reasonable doubt whether the arsenic so administered was in fact the cause of his death". A re-examination of her case resulted in her release in 1904 and she returned to her native America where she died in 1941 at the age of 79. Amongst her papers was found a magazine article about how to use arsenic from fly-paper as a beauty treatment.

As recently as 2010, a Lakhvir Singh, a mother of three from west London, was convicted at the Old Bailey, of poisoning the curry she had served up to her ex-lover and the new girlfriend he had chosen to marry. He died. She had travelled to India to obtain aconite, known as the 'queen of poisons'. Aconite contains powerful alkaloids, attacking the nervous system. Despite it being lethal, it is still contained within homeopathic preparations and some traditional Chinese herbal medicines.

All parts of the yew tree, except the scarlet aril (berry) are highly toxic, owing to the presence of taxine alkaloids, which are cardio toxic. Management of yew poisoning is merely supportive as no antidote exists. Castor oil seeds contain ricin and the decorative plant Oleander is highly toxic. There is a persisting but unsubstantiated story of a group of individuals who used oleander twigs as kebab sticks and how they all died, even though they had only eaten the meat. It is said that all fungi are edible but some, you only eat once! The cherry laurel tree, sometimes used to create hedges, can be confused with the bay tree, and used in cooking. The leaves and fruit pips are capable of releasing cyanide, giving them the characteristic bitter almond smell. Roughly 1.5% cyanogenic glycosides are present in the leaves, which, when macerated, release glucose, hydrogen cyanide and benzaldehyde. It is generally advised that clippings and chippings should be dealt with in the open air and not transported in cars and vans to the local tip.

Nothing could be more natural than the passage of time as our planet orbits the sun giving the rhythm of day and night. However, the recording of time was "local" prior to the railway age and the need for a standard time to facilitate train timetables. Once upon a time a small town had two public clocks, one on the church and the other outside the clockmaker's shop. All the citizens took their cue from these clocks which always told the same time but were wrong! The Sexton set the church clock each day at noon with reference to the clock maker's instrument without knowing that the clockmaker had set his time earlier from that of the church!

The success of Nelson's navy was in part due to two factors. Superior navigation resulted from the development of the chronometer which allowed accurate longitude to be established at sea. Superior speed came from the practise of copper-bottoming the ships to discourage barnacles from attaching themselves and adding a drag effect. Much of the copper ore was mined and smelted near Swansea.

CHAPTER NINE

The Macabre

Death lurks and smirks at us all our lives. The only decent response is to smile nicely when the time comes. From the first days in medical school, doctors are exposed to death. Initially, these are cadavers for dissection, with progression through clinical studies, revealing the grim reality of death in hospital. In my younger days, few people died peaceful deaths in hospital. Death was inevitably preceded by the usually futile ritual of cardiopulmonary resuscitation. This was often accompanied by inappropriate treatment. The use of DNA CPR (do not attempt cardio-pulmonary resuscitation) notices is often the correct medicine but is can be misinterpreted by relatives as a negative act.

The use of Cardio-Pulmonary Resuscitation

Contrary to popular opinion, (often gleaned from TV medical soap operas), successful resuscitation after cardiac arrest is much less than 50% in those of middle age, with little co-morbidity. Over 75 years of age, in the presence of multiple co-morbidities, success is vanishingly small, often very short-lived (minutes/hours/days) and usually accompanied by serious brain damage, especially if cerebrovascular disease co-exists. If attempted, it is almost always futile and can turn a peaceful impending death into a distressing drama. Whether to attempt it or not, is ultimately a medical decision. It is best practice to discuss matters with the patient or next of kin (if the patient lacks capacity) and inform them of the reasons why a DNAR order is appropriate. Doctors are under no obligation to perform futile treatments which might not be in the patient's best interests. Neither the patient nor next of kin can demand resuscitation if it is medically inappropriate.

A more positive spin, achieving the same result, is to declare an AND (Allow Natural Death) notice. The use of the Liverpool Care Pathway dramatically improved the experiences of dying patients and their relatives.

The use of "Care of the dying Pathways"

The Liverpool Care Pathway (LCP) was developed for widespread use, from the experiences of those dealing with terminally ill patients in hospices. It provided a clear concise set of guidelines to ensure that dying patients did not suffer through mismanagement and pointless over-treatment. Prior to 2013, these pathways were commonly used when it was apparent that the life of a patient was drawing to a close. They had Government backing and such pathways enshrined the best principles of practice, to ensure that death was as peaceful as possible, by concentrating on symptom relief and discouraging irrelevant medical actions. Following a furore of media attention during 2013, the Government withdrew its backing. Where these pathways had "bad press", it was usually the case that they were either inappropriately commenced, or poorly delivered, or done without informing the next of kin. It was the implementation of the pathways, not their principles, which were criticised. Recent polls have revealed that a substantial majority of doctors would still wish for their own terminal care to be delivered according to the principles of these pathways. They do not hasten death but they do not prolong the process of dying either. Those principles of good end of life care still apply, are used regularly and are considered to represent "best practice". All death causes upset to family members and although death from a long illness is often anticipated, it is sometimes not actually expected as quickly as often happens. This can cause a serious mismatch of expectations between professionals and family. Sometimes delaying the implementation of care pathway principles for a few days allows time for views to converge but the interest of the patient must always come first. Any delays primarily for the benefit of family should only be done if not detrimental to the patient's best interest.

The human body starts to decompose some four minutes after death. Rigor mortis results from the chemical effects on the muscles; by the lactate and phosphate produced from the breakdown of the transmitter ATP. The first muscles to be affected are the erector pili, which produces the gooseflesh. The small facial muscles are affected within five hours, followed by the arms before ten hours and then the trunk and the legs by twelve hours. Rigor remains, and then softens between twenty-four and thirty-six hours. Cadaveric spasm is a marked rigor, associated with violent or emotional deaths. Body fluids tend to drain under gravity, producing hypostasis, which has its onset within an hour and is maximal maximum at five hours. Under natural circumstances but dependent upon temperature of the surroundings, the body starts to cool and putrefy. Some green discolouration in the flanks becomes noticeable between thirty-six and forty-eight hours, marbling of the veins between seventy-two and ninety-six hours and swelling of the body occurs within five to six days. The common bluebottle, of species calliphora, lays its eggs in daylight in soft areas of the corpse, around the eyes, mouth and wounds. The resulting maggots pass through a number of stages, before pupating. The bluebottles are initially attracted to corpses by the characteristic smell of recent death. {Hawthorn blossom, according to folk-lore, brings bad luck if brought into the house. It has a heavy complex scent due to the presence of triethylamine which is also one of the first chemicals produced by a corpse. (Triethylamine also smells like semen)} There are beetles, which feed upon maggots. To gain a maximum feast, they have adapted to be attracted by the smell of a body, some six to seven days old, which occurs around the time when the maggots have fattened up. As they become close to pupation, the final stage of maggot leaves the corpse – an evolutionary adaptation to avoid the approaching beetles. They tend to move in a southerly direction (in the northern hemisphere), before resting and pupating, so the maggots effectively head off and can travel surprisingly long distances in warm weather at the same time that the beetles approach. It is normally some ten days before the swarm of bluebottles, buzzing around net curtains and exiting the house through the letter box, alerts the neighbours and then the police to the presence of a dead body within.

Much has been learned about the natural history of decay under varied circumstances from the work of Professor Bass at the Body Farm in Tennessee. However, the natural speed of decay of corpses, which have received active treatment, appears to be different. This is of great concern to cemetery directors, who find that the corpses are not decomposing fast enough. There are a number of theories:

- That corpses are no longer put on show for a few days. This allowed bacteria and egg laying flies to settle on the corpse, speeding up decomposition.
- Too much humidity can turn the body fat into a soapy substance, known as adipocere or grave wax.
- There may be a shortage of worms in the ground.
- Antibiotics prescribed before death may further influence the bacterial load.
- Most modern coffins are made from chipboard, covered with paper printed to look like oak or mahogany. The chipboard is manufactured using formaldehyde, which may act as a preservative. Because of the shortage of land, this has been a major problem in Venice and they have been experimenting with adding liquid and powdered enzymes to corpses, prior to burial

The rise in obesity has resulted in larger coffins, some of which take up the space of two plots and have to be interned with the help of a crane. The oversized corpses have fuelled a change in coffin design, with rectangular caskets and cigar shaped coffins growing in popularity, above the traditional tapered design, which is widest at the shoulders. Some of these coffins are too large to fit inside a hearse. To bury a large person of thirty stone, the coffin is not only heavy but has the appearance of a small wardrobe; too heavy to be lowered by hand and requiring mechanical devices at the graveside.

Hygienic disposal of corpses to prevent disease and water contamination has been practised for millennia but the mode of disposal has evolved according to religious rites. Traditionally, and in conjunction with bacterial putrefaction and maggot consumption, carrion feeders played a vital role. Vultures in particular historically played an important role as the optimal natural animal disposal system because a vulture's metabolism is a true "dead-end" for pathogens. Wild dogs, wild cats and rats can easily become carriers of diseases including anthrax, rabies, and plague.

Vultures still have a crucial role in the death rituals of the Zoroastrian Parsees of Mumbai. There are however problems! The religion is interesting and outlined in detail in the following article:

Contractor, Dinshaw and Hutoxy. "Zoroastrianism: History, Beliefs, and Practices." Quest 91.1 (JANUARY – FEBRUARY 2003):4-9.

I learnt the basic background on holiday in India and expand as below.

Zoroaster, known as (the shining light) Zarathustra by the Greeks, was the Persian prophet upon whose teachings the ancient religion of Zoroastrianism is based. He was probably born around 1500 BC. Zoroastrianism is now the smallest of the major religions of the world. With roots in the ancient beliefs which spawned the religions of India, it was the first of the world's religions to be founded by an inspired and reforming prophet. It also influenced the religions of Judaism, Christianity, and Islam based upon the common threads within the

Old Testament. Zoroastrianism was the first religion to conceptualise the following:-

- A cosmic struggle between good and evil
- The primacy of ethical choice in human life
- Monotheism
- A heavenly hierarchy of spirits such as angels and archangels which mediate between God and humanity
- A judgment for each individual after death
- The coming of a Messiah at the end of this creation
- A final apocalypse culminating in the triumph of Good over evil.

In Zoroastrianism Ahura Mazda, is the "Wise Lord, God and the head of the universe" From him came all life. Followers aim to have good thoughts, good words and resultant good deeds. Fire is the major symbol in Zoroastrianism and has a central role in the most important religious ceremonies, being the supreme symbol of God and the divine Life. Ahura Mazda is described in the scriptures as "full of lustre, full of glory," and as such his creations fire, sun, stars, and light in general are revered as symbolising the divine spark of inner light which is present in us all. Fire is also a physical representation of the illuminated mind.

The Zoroastrian place of worship is the fire temple within which an eternal flame is kept burning with sandalwood and frankincense. The fire temples are open only to Zoroastrians. The first fire to be lit upon an altar is said to have been brought down from heaven by Zoroaster with a rod.

The religion thrived in Persia until 641 A.D, when the Arabs invaded and established Islam therein as the belief of choice. The new rulers gave the local population a tough time imposing three choices upon them. The preferred option was conversion to Islam. Alternatives were the payment of a heavy tax (Jizya) imposed on nonbelievers or death. The Arabs on-going persecution of the Zoroastrians made day-to-day life very difficult for those who refused to convert. {As Macmillan was to observe 1300 years later and we have seen ourselves in later years, no Middle Eastern ruler is so bad that his replacement cannot turn out to be worse}.

Consequently, in 936 A.D., a group of Zoroastrians from the town of Sanjan in the Khorasan Province of Iran made their way south to the port of Hormuz on the Persian Gulf and set sail for India. They wandered in slow transit for almost twenty years before making final landfall on the western coast of Gujarat where they were granted sanctuary. After they settled in India, fire was again brought down from heaven by lightning to create the sacred symbol of Ahura Mazda.

These immigrants to India became known as the Parsees (those from the Persian province of Pars). The Parsees prospered in Gujarat and later on began to spread out to other parts of India including Bombay (Mumbai) where they particularly excelled and prospered after British rule was established. 45,000 of India's 61,000 Parsee Zoroastrians currently live in Mumbai.

Zoroastrianism places great emphasis on purity and not defiling any of the sacred elements of Ahura

Mazda's creation. Earth, Fire, and Water are the key sacred elements therefore burial at sea, cremation and burial in the earth are sacrilegious acts. Instead, dead bodies were taken to a Tower of Silence, stripped naked, and laid out under the sun, where scores of vultures serving as messengers between heaven and earth devoured them within hours and liberated the soul. At the present time, there is a problem because a shortage of vultures means that the Parsee Indians, deprived of their celestial intermediaries, have been obliged to alter these ancient customs for reasons of hygiene, since bodies now take six months to disappear. The Tower of Silence in Mumbai is situated in the very affluent suburb of Malabar hill. Although it remains out of sight it lies within a 54-acre plot of greenery on the potential real estate goldmine of Doongerwadi – Imagine how this would go down in Manhattan or Mayfair!

Nine species of vulture live in India with most currently in danger of extinction. In the 1980s there were as many as 80 million white-rumped vultures (*Gyps bengalensis*) when it was the most numerous species of raptor in the world. Today, however, its population numbers only several thousand. The vulture population had been seeing a slow but steady decline due to habitat destruction but the current crisis is the result of them being poisoned by the anti-inflammatory painkiller drug Diclofenac given to animals. This is highly toxic to the vultures who also feed on animal carcases – especially cows. Hindus do not eat cows, which they consider sacred. {When one of the estimated 500 million head of cattle in India dies, it is not eaten by humans, but left in situ for the vultures}. Cows are used for milk products and as very important beasts of burden. Diclofenac was used to treat the symptoms of inflammation, fevers and/or pain to keep the animal active. The drug was banned in May 2006, but by then it had decimated 95% of the vulture population. The replacement drug Meloxicam was quickly developed. It treats cattle the same way as Diclofenac, but is harmless to vultures. Despite this vulture populations have continued to decline in India at a rate of between 20% and 40% each year since 2007. The Towers of Silence in Mumbai have found an alternative by using powerful solar concentrators which desiccate the corpses over days rather than in the hours that a hungry flock of vultures accomplished. This method still keeps to Zarathushtra's injunction not to defile the elements. The solar-concentrator option has also retained the religious relevance of Doongerwadi which means that redevelopment of the site is unlikely for the time being.

Most people are currently cremated in the UK but standard crematoria, with chambers of thirty-five inches, across cannot cope with the obese. Newer ones are being installed in some crematoria at forty-three inches wide. The funeral industry is said to be the second biggest source of pollution, after fossil fuel fired power stations. One council was heavily criticised for planning to warm the municipal swimming pool with the excess heat generated by the incinerator at the nearby crematorium. A serious problem arises from the emission of mercury when teeth containing amalgam fillings are burnt. Attempts are made to deal with this at conventional gas cremators with filters in the chimneys; however, these are not 100% effective and, as a consequence, 19% of airborne mercury is attributed to crematoria. Even with better filtration, this level is set to rise as the number of people dying with their own teeth intact increases. The obvious answer to the problem is to remove either the fillings or the teeth containing them. Cardiac pacemakers must be removed before cremation. In the UK use of cremation as a means of disposal is a relatively recent phenomenon with an interesting history going back less than 150 years. It all began in 1883 in the small town of Llantrisant, in the Rhondda northwest of Cardiff where the eccentric eighty-year-old Welshman and self-styled druid Dr William Price lived. Today Llantrisant is best known as the home of the Royal Mint from which it has acquired the unfair soubriquet "The hole with the mint." The ancient Druids of pre-Christian Britain were the priests, teachers, political advisors, healers and arbiters to the Celtic tribes. Their actual beliefs and practices are obscured by lack of any of their contemporaneous written records. They were eliminated by the Romans and all we really know from Pliny the elder is that oak and mistletoe played significant roles. The Celtic revival of the 18th and 19th centuries led to neo-druidism in which beliefs and rituals evolved from myth and fantasy.

In any event by 1883 Price had taken to wearing fancy costume involving a scarlet waistcoat and fox-skin headpiece and often paraded through the town carrying a blazing torch and a druid's crescent moon as symbols of his beliefs. He lived with his housekeeper who was nearly sixty years his junior with whom he fathered a child named Iesu Grist (Jesus Christ). The child sadly died at the age of five months. Dr Price was devastated.

On the following Sunday, he took the body to a hilltop above Llantrisant where in full view of the nearby chapel he attempted to cremate the body using paraffin. An angry crowd of locals dragged the body from the pyre and nearly killed Price in the process. The police became involved. An autopsy was hastily performed on Iesu's body and concluded that the child had died of natural causes. Price could not therefore be charged with infanticide. However, he was tried in Cardiff for performing cremation rather than a burial. The police believed this to be an illegal act.

Price successfully argued that while the law did not state that cremation was legal, it also did not state that it was illegal. The judge, Mr. Justice Stephen, agreed. On 14 March, he was finally able to give his son a cremation in a neo druidic ceremony. In 1885 the first official cremation took place at Woking, and ten cremations are recorded as being performed in the following year. In 1892 a crematorium opened in Manchester followed by one in Glasgow in 1895 and one in Liverpool in 1896. The case's legal precedent, together with the activities of the newly founded Cremation Society of Great Britain, led to legislation. The Cremation Act 1902 was an Act of Parliament which applied to England and Wales, and Scotland, but not to Ireland. It came into effect on 1 April 1903. The Act has since been heavily amended, but remains in force. The major purpose of the Act was to allow burial authorities to establish crematoria. No crematorium built could be closer than fifty yards to any public highway, or in the consecrated area of a burial ground. It could not be built within two hundred yards of any dwelling house without the written consent of the owner, lessee and occupier, and the act was not to be interpreted to "authorise the burial authority or any person to create or permit a nuisance". Later versions of the Act were used to outlaw open air cremations using funeral pyres, although in 2010 the Court of Appeal ruled this practice to be legal under certain circumstances.

The Secretary of State created regulations for the maintenance and inspection of crematoria, the circumstances in which they could be used, and the creation of a register of such burnings. All statutory provisions relating to the use of burial registers as evidence were to apply to these registers.

Any breach of these regulations, or burning of human remains outside of the provisions of the Act, would be liable, on summary conviction, to a penalty of up to fifty pounds. Any person found guilty of wilfully making any false representations in order to procure the burning of human remains would be liable to imprisonment with or without hard labour for up to two years; and any person found guilty of attempting to conceal an offence by attempting to procure the burning of human remains would be liable to imprisonment with or without hard labour for up to five years.

Open air funeral pyres were made illegal in Britain by the 1930 amendment to the Cremation Act. Prior to this, but after the 1902 Act, open air cremations had occurred in limited numbers including those for Hindu and Sikh soldiers killed in WW 1 who were cremated in Brighton. The last legal open air pyre is believed to have occurred in 1934, when the British Government gave special permission to Nepal's ambassador to cremate his wife outdoors in Surrey.

In 2006, Davender Ghai, a British citizen and devout Hindu who had arrived from Kenya in 1958, launched a judicial review of the Act after Newcastle-upon-Tyne City Council refused him a permit to conduct open air cremations in Britain in accordance with Hindu religious practices. He had been campaigning for open air funerals for people of any faith, arguing there was significant demand from the increasingly aging British Hindu and Sikh communities who, due to the restrictions of the Act, often flew bodies of their relatives abroad for cremation. In July 2006, believing the law did not prohibit pyres, Mr. Ghai organised the open-air cremation of Rajpal Mehat, an Indian-born Sikh illegal immigrant, who was found drowned in a London canal. Subsequent delays in identification meant the body was not fit to be repatriated, and Mehat's relatives asked Ghai to organise the ceremony in accordance with their beliefs. The ceremony, held in a field in Northumbria, was Britain's first open air cremation since 1934. Informed prior to the ceremony, local police initially allowed it to take place, but then said it had been illegal. The Crown Prosecution Service agreed, but ruled a prosecution would not be in the public interest. Shortly afterwards, Ghai launched his judicial review to seek clarification of the law and the council's refusal under the Act. In February 2010 the Court of Appeal ruled that, as long as open air pyres took place within a structure of some sort, that the practice would be legal under the existing Act, although there were outstanding planning and environmental regulatory issues to be settled before pyres would actually be possible.

A number of firms are experimenting with alternatives to cremation. These include resonation, involving alkaline hydrolysis – heating and treating the body, so it decomposes quickly, leaving just bone ash and a small amount of liquid. An alternative process, promession, involves freezing the remains in liquid nitrogen before they are mechanically shattered and dried into an organic powder. Once buried in a shallow grave within a cemetery or natural burial park, the remains are converted into soil within a year.

There is confusion as to where, when and how ashes may be scattered. Many people have a preference to scatter them at beauty spots, with the Snowdonia National Park consistently warning about the impact ashes can have on the environment. Wardens at Windermere in the Lake District National Park have indicated that it is acceptable to scatter ashes in the lake but not to throw whole urns into the water. The ashes must be scattered loose. One enterprising firm (www.ashesintoglass.co.uk) advertises turning cremation ashes into glass, which can be moulded into jewellery or various objects and kept for posterity. One Xmas my wife received one of those robot cleaners which have a docking station and according to the timings set, come out to clean automatically. We chuckled on remembering an episode from the BBC mystery crime series "Jonathan Creek." Someone's ashes were spilled on the carpet just before the relative went out for an appointment. They were left in situ to be gathered up upon return. They vanished but were eventually found in the robot having been "hoovered up."

The phenomenon of grave rage is a growing concern, with grieving families falling out over tributes, such as teddy bears, flowers and even food left at the grave. Families from different cultures celebrate the death in different ways and cemeteries have to give clear guidance on items that might be a hazard, such as candles, or food which might attract vermin. Squirrels are particularly partial to eating carnations and chrysanthemums because of their high sugar content and in search of these, spread mess far and wide. Other flowers are being suggested and squirrel repellent is being discretely sprayed. Wind chimes, cellophane wrapping around flowers and stuffed animals in plastic bags can also prove particularly irritant to visitors. I heard of someone whose wish was to be buried with his mobile phone switched on in his pocket and was to be rung, to check that he was really dead, before the coffin was finally lowered. It is always advisable to turn your mobile phone off if attending the graveside ceremony. One mourner was extremely embarrassed when his handset went off; breaking the silence, with the ringtone of the Bee Gee's hit 'Staying Alive'. Favourite tunes, played at cremations, have included 'Smoke Gets in Your Eyes', 'Wish Me Luck as You Wave Me Goodbye', Elvis Presley's 'Return to Sender', 'Stairway to Heaven', 'Another One Bites the Dust', 'Ring of Fire' and 'Nellie the Elephant Packed Her Trunk'. One family requested the 'Robin Hood' theme, meaning the slow dirge 'Everything I do, I do it for you'. Unintentionally, the music played was from the 1960s television version, 'Robin Hood, Robin Hood, riding through the Glen'.

The Vietnamese have a curious ritual following death. The corpse is buried in a rough grave, often on raised dry ground in the paddy field, for some three years. Thereafter, the responsibility of the eldest son is to dig up the corpse, scrape off any remaining flesh and rearrange the bones in a much smaller coffin, which is then reburied in a more permanent mausoleum. One man in Vietnam made the papers. He dug up his wife's body and slept beside it for five years, because he wished to hug her every night in bed. He opened his wife's grave a year after she was buried and moulded clay around her remains.

Burial at sea was a method hypothetically suggested by the then Medical Officer of Health for Liverpool, Dr Duncan Dolton, in which unburied bodies could be buried at sea during any extended strike by the gravediggers' union during the 1978-9 Winter of Discontent. British Naval burials at sea of the 18th and

19th century involved sewing the deceased in sailcloth, weighted with cannonballs, with the last stitch passing through the nose to wake any who were merely comatose.

Today, the rules for burial at sea are stringent in the United Kingdom. Cremated remains may be scattered freely at sea, but a burial must be made in a coffin meeting regulatory requirements and in one of three locations: off the Needles on the Isle of Wight; between Hastings and Newhaven on the south east coast; or off Tynemouth, North Tyneside. Permission may also be sought for the use of alternative sites. Bodies cannot be embalmed and must be clad in biodegradable material ("commensurate with modesty"); coffins must be made of softwood and may not have plastic, zinc, copper, or lead fittings. British regulators are preoccupied with preventing bodies from washing up on shore or getting snagged in fishing equipment. They require coffins to be heavily weighted and drilled with 40 to 50 holes. Though it is rare, bodies do occasionally resurface. Just in case, each body must have an ID tag locked around its neck.

Research into underwater decomposition using the bodies of various mammals concluded that a body and a shroud on the sea floor should completely disintegrate within three to six months. Forensic experts consider that after two days in the water, most bodies are "unrecognizable."

The Environment Agency says that no laws prevent one person being buried in their own garden, but an authorisation form must be filled in, since decomposing corpses can pose a health risk to the living. A garden grave must be situated more than 10 metres from standing water, at least 50 metres away from a drinking water source, and be deep enough to dissuade foxes from digging up the dearly departed. It is also necessary to record the whereabouts of the grave and include this in the deeds of the property. More than one grave requires the garden to be registered as a cemetery.

The unfamiliarity of the general public with death, can lead to some seemingly bizarre actions. One son, who had taken his elderly mother out for the day in her wheelchair, found that she had died. He fluffed her up and took her home on the bus. Unfortunately for him, her lack of life was apparent to other passengers and the police were called. Some years ago, two ladies tried to take the body of their dead elderly relation onto an Easy Jet flight, at John Lennon Airport, smuggled in a wheelchair. They had managed to get him to the airport in a taxi. His death was all too apparent to the security staff and the police were called. The two ladies were arrested on suspicion of failing to give notification of death. They had decided to try and board the flight, rather than pay up to six thousand pounds in repatriation fees for the body. Hospitals have faced legal actions after they have released the wrong body. In one particularly sad case, a lady who wished to be buried with her family was cremated and in another case, bodies were released to the wrong families. A classic Rolls-Royce hearse being used in Teeside had to be hot-wired in order to get to the cemetery after a rival undertaker stole the keys whilst it was parked outside a church. The culprit received a community sentence and the victim compensated.

Inscriptions on tomb stones, especially the older ones, provide a hidden code. A half column on a grave indicates a life cut short, whereas the skull and skeleton motifs are there as a reference to the belief in the resurrection of the body and soul on the day of judgement. Symbolic flames on tomb stones represent the hope of eternal life and the promise to remember the dead forever. The laurel wreath and its persisting green leaves is a reference to an everlasting soul. Those wreaths which are a complete circle indicate a life lived to the full, whereas, an incomplete horse shoe shape suggest that death has come too soon. A yew tree within the graveyard symbolises eternal life, whereas the smell of the leaves was thought in medieval times to be capable of covering up the smell of dead bodies, which had been unceremoniously piled in open common graves. The leaves themselves, if eaten, would poison any sheep that strayed in. The coiled snake biting its own tail speaks of the hope of rejuvenation and a whale on a tombstone comes from the story of Jonah, who, having been swallowed by a whale, re-emerged some three days later. This is a reference to a necessary period in purgatory for minor sins. An unusual tomb stands on Rodney Street in Liverpool. It is that of a wealthy Victorian Railway Engineer, by the name of Will Mackenzie, whose tomb is a pyramid. It is alleged that he once played the devil in a game of poker, gambling his soul. He of course lost and now sits in that tomb with a winning hand of cards, strapped to his chest, to cheat the devil.

The Halifax gibbet, referred to earlier, which was the precursor of the guillotine, came to the attention of a Scottish Earl, James Douglas, who attended an execution in Halifax in the sixteenth century. Upon his return to Edinburgh, he had a similar instrument made for use in the Scottish capital. It was this machine that caught the imagination of Dr Guillotine at the beginning of the

French revolution. Through trial and error, the instrument was gradually refined and the edge of the blade changed from the original crescent shaped blade, to that of the 45° angle. By 1792, it had reached its final form, which remained in use until the 1970s. The founder of modern chemistry, Antoine Lavoisier, was guillotined during the revolutionary reign of terror for allegedly adulterating the tobacco supply. He planned to deliberately blink for as long as possible after decapitation as an experiment. His friends observed him blinking for 15 seconds. By the early 1900s, some doctors were concerned that the guillotine was not quite such a humane method of execution, as had hitherto been believed. Experiments were performed, which were subsequently published in the 1906 Archives D'Anthropologie Criminelle. A Dr Marcoux had groomed a subject due for execution. He closely observed the events following decapitation. The head fortuitously had fallen upright into the basket and there was little haemorrhage from the neck. It was noted that the muscles of the lips and eyelids twitched and contracted for several seconds following decapitation and then the eyelids half closed. However, the head responded to the voice of Dr Marcoux by the eyelids opening and then the pupils turning slightly upward, focusing themselves upon the doctor and holding his gaze for some ten to fifteen seconds. From further changes in facial expressions suggesting agony, together with eye movements and movements of the lips suggesting the wish to speak, Dr Marcoux was of the opinion that the brain was still alive for some minutes after decapitation. Similar observations were subsequently recorded by other medical practitioners; the practical importance of this has proven of use when considering how long the brain can survive after cardiac arrest.

An acquaintance of mine told me a sad story, about a family friend. He was a recently retired doctor, in his 60s, whose wife had sadly died. He was fit and active and fairly adventurous. He decided to spend some six months of 1974 cycling around Europe. His arrangements were somewhat loose and he made no specific commitment to stay in communication. He left his hometown in Yorkshire, aiming to cycle to Dover, catch the ferry and take matters day-by-day. His family were not really expecting him to return until the autumn and were not unduly surprised at the lack of post cards. However, when he failed to return by Christmas, with still no communication, he was listed by the police as an official missing person and his description circulated to Interpol. A year passed, with still no news. His body was eventually discovered, hidden by heavy undergrowth, in a small valley at the side of a steep hill, near Dover. It was assumed that, whilst riding downhill, he had been sideswiped by a truck, pitched over the low barrier and ended up in undergrowth, to be left undiscovered.

An unusual case in Wallasey in 2010, involved the death of a 95-year-old lady at home. She lived with her daughter and granddaughter. She occupied the small bedroom in the house and probably died of natural causes. However, neither the daughter nor granddaughter reported the death. She had probably died around Christmas time but the corpse was not discovered until August. They had simply closed the door and turned off the central heating in that room. It was only in the summer months when neighbours became concerned about persisting bluebottles visible through the windows that police were alerted. The corpse was in an advanced stage of decomposition and pathologists were unable to identify any specific cause of death. The couple were charged with, and both pleaded guilty to, leaving the corpse unburied. They also admitted to cashing in her state pension. On a lighter note, a local butcher put a large sign in his window, which read 'Watership Down, you have read the book; you have seen the film, now eat the cast'. He was persuaded to take down the sign, within a few hours.

Sadly, far too many people who wish to die at home, in fact die in hospital. The hospital deathbed scene is fairly grim, for both patient and relatives. The ideal death is the 'goldilocks' death, neither too fast, nor too slow. If death occurs too quickly, there is little time for family to come to terms with matters. Cause of death is often uncertain and this results in a coroner's post mortem and sometimes an inquest. The prolonged death causes enormous family tensions. The situation is often that grown up children, coming from all parts of the UK and sometimes from abroad, have gathered around the hospital bed, to pay their last respects. Their spouses and sometimes their children will also be in attendance. These individuals may not have spent much time together for forty years and suddenly, they are put into high tension situations, where lack of sleep and lack of privacy can contribute to the general upset of seeing a loved one about to die. It is surprisingly common for family rows to breakout if the deathbed scene drags out for more than seventy-two hours. No one wishes to be seen to be the first to go for a break or a rest and few dare to return to their own homes, before the inevitable outcome. Lack of food and lack of sleep contribute to tiredness, which merely exacerbates the emotional cauldron. Doctors and nurses get caught in the crossfire and can be accused of negligence. It has been said that the death of George V was advanced, such that his death occurred in a timely manner so that it could be announced in the morning papers, rather than in the evening papers.

CHAPTER TEN

Things Military

The Territorial Army (TA) came into existence on the 1st April 1908. It was created by merger of the Yeomanry (a volunteer Calvary force, formed at the time of the French revolution, to maintain order) with the Volunteers. Thereafter, it had an illustrious record, providing the backbone for expansion of UK land forces, when the need arose. As Churchill observed, TA volunteers were "twice a citizen". He also thought that nothing in life is so exhilarating as to be shot at without result.

I received my commission as Captain, in December 1980. This was the time of the Russian occupation of Afghanistan and global tensions were rising. Motivations for volunteering and joining the Territorial Army are as diverse as the individuals it attracts. Some use it as a stepping stone to joining the regular forces; some join for the social life but most join for adventure and the spirit of comradeship which it engenders. A handful of individuals join solely for the altruistic motive of serving their country, but for most people there is a mixture of reasons. The commitment is normally one evening per week, a weekend a month and a two week annual camp. Many attend for training on most Sundays of the year.

The Territorial Army was designed to be mobilised on mass in the 1980s, in the event of Russian land forces crossing the inner German border and advancing westwards against the NATO alliance. Being medical, I joined the local 208 General Hospital Unit. This was a unit designed to set up a rather static large general hospital unit to deal with mass casualties, after they had been processed through field ambulances and dressing stations and field hospitals. It was top-heavy with professionals with diverse medical skills and most were commissioned. The TA provided military training on the basis that anyone wearing a uniform was a soldier first and a professional second. There was a symbiotic relationship between these civilians and the regular army. The army benefited considerably from their diverse civilian skills acquired from all walks of life and individuals who joined received top quality training in management and administration from the army. Civilian employers benefited from these skills acquired by allowing people to volunteer. For the most part, the regular army recruits soldiers and officers at a relatively young age and provides the training. By contrast, the TA recruit is usually much older, with wider experience of life and often having specific skills and qualifications.

The medical unit was not exclusively comprised of doctors, nurses and medical orderlies. We had detachments from the REME (Royal Electrical and Mechanical Engineers), the Catering corps, the Pay corps, drivers and weapons specialists. A unit such as ours was primarily surgically orientated, but physicians such as myself had a major role in potential management of medical casualties from disease or chemical warfare.

One routine role for all medical officers was to perform medical examinations on new recruits. For the most part, they were generally fit people whose ability to run and march had already been assessed. However, on one occasion, I was tasked with doing twenty routine assessments in a morning. I made a very cursory abdominal examination on one recruit, only to find an enormous spleen. When quizzed, he denied all knowledge. I made further enquiries of his general practitioner, to find that he had a glycogen storage disease, a genetic condition, which had been diagnosed in infancy. He was clearly unfit for medical service, largely because a spleen of that size could easily rupture and cause death from relatively minor injury. I am not sure what his motives for joining were but I suspect they may not have been entirely honourable.

Many older sergeants and officers had served in theatres of war, as national servicemen. Conflicts in Aden and Cyprus had been particularly harrowing for young soldiers. During the late 1950s, Greek-Cypriot terrorists mounted regular ambushes on British troops. The main central avenue of Nicosia, Ledra Street, was known as 'murder mile' because of the number of lives claimed by assassins. One of our sergeants had been there as a national serviceman. His platoon was comprised of a mixture of ordinary young men, some thugs and some 'mummy's boys', who were mutually suspicious of one another. He told me that their officer had a novel way of getting this group to bond. He dumped them in the middle of Ledra Street, in full uniform, telling them to protect each other and return to camp in two hours. Under the common threat, they bonded rapidly and by the time they returned to camp, the boys had grown up.

The two week camps were an excellent way of bonding with and getting to know the whole unit membership. The camp was usually structured around a five day exercise, with the remaining time being spent on general administration and more general training. Camps were mostly held in the UK but occasionally, every two years, abroad. Belgium and Germany were common destinations. During one such exercise, a visiting General was mingling with the troops and making light conversation. He asked one medical orderly what he did in civilian life. His response was 'a government artist Sir'. The General enquired further, explaining that he thought that must be an interesting job, with the further comment, 'what do you actually do'? The response was 'I draw the dole'.

On a large military base in the north of England, I was tasked with moving a platoon a mile across country, unseen. Not only did I fail miserably but made the mistake of straying into the territory of a completely unrelated exercise being held by some regular troops. We were ambushed with thunder flashes, bright lights and the firing of thousands of blank rounds. We were all captured. As the officer, I was given special interrogation. I was tied to a chair and whilst not actually seriously physically abused, was certainly roughed up.

On a weekend exercise, we had set up a general hospital unit, designed to test our ability to process casualties. This was a freezing cold February; with the exercise starting late on Friday night and continuing through to Sunday lunch time. Our 'casualties' were volunteer army cadets and those from the local CCF. They had been made up to look like casualties elsewhere and had been bussed into us, on lorries, for processing. By midnight, the roads had become dangerously icy and for health and safety reasons, it was decided to pause the exercise overnight. These young lads, who were mostly under the age of seventeen, were held in our makeshift tented wards. We had not been fully equipped with blankets and there was little in the way of heating for the tents and what there was proved inadequate for purpose. By 4 am, most of these lads were cold and miserable and in danger of getting actual hypothermia. One of their warrant officers came up with the ideal solution. He arranged for a nearby field to be floodlit, mustered his cadets and ran them around the field, for the two hours until 6 am, in order for them to keep warm. In the meantime, the field kitchen had prepared double rations. About 6.30 am, there was the call for 'grub up'. There was a stampede of young cadets, grabbing handfuls of bread from loaves and filling their mess tins with as much as could be crammed in. I have never seen anyone eat so much, so quickly. Come dawn, the exercise was resumed. The RAF had provided helicopters to evacuate the casualties onwards. In reality, they were to be flown back to the start position and sent through again and again. The helicopters, which the RAF had provided, were designed to strap six casualties on stretchers into the space. The stretchers were suspended in tiers of three, one on each side, and the casualties were supposed to be strapped securely into the stretcher, which, in turn was supposed to be securely fastened to the suspension webbing in the helicopter. When one of these helicopters banked steeply, one of these young lads became detached from his harness and was seen clinging on for grim death to the side of his stretcher, with his legs hanging out of the open helicopter side door, until it resumed a more levelled flight. To add insult to injury, before departure, they were paraded. Their warrant officer checked who had not paid their two pounds for this wonderful experience.

At one annual camp, where again we were processing casualties, they were comprised of regular troops. During a lull in the proceedings, it was suggested that we get some of our 'casualties' to leg it over to the cook house and get an urn full of tea. Two were duly dispatched and returned in a timely manner. They came back with a large tea urn, the size of a small beer keg, with a tap at the base. The tea was unremarkable but weaker than usual. In these urns, the tea leaves were contained within a perforated metal canister, accessed from the top. To try and make the tea a little stronger, someone opened up the top to mash the tea leaves around. He was somewhat surprised to find that there was no tea actually in the canister. Someone had forgotten to add it but had added the water. The tea we were in fact drinking had come entirely from the staining on the inside of the urn, from previous generations of use.

At annual camp, messing arrangements were usually very comfortable. Officers generally paid extra money to augment the rations and we lived very well. Breakfast was usually fully cooked, as was lunch and a sumptuous dinner in the evening. There would always be some formal dinners, usually with speeches. Because of the predominance of female officers from the nursing corps, our mess was relatively well-behaved. It was, however, a pleasure to be invited to dine at a regular army mess and to experience the sort of behaviour which one thought one had left behind at school. A specialty of an artillery mess was firing homemade mortars at the end of the meal. The essential equipment appeared to be a box of matches and an empty large cigar tube. Firstly, the heads of the full box of matches were detached and packed into the base of the cigar tube. A suitable light but nonlethal missile was then added and the whole lot wadded tightly into the base of the tube and then held firmly into position with some thick mashed potato or chewed banana. The mortar was then carefully positioned and the base heated by means of a cigarette lighter. In due course, the match heads therein would ignite and the missile be discharged with a suitable spray of potato or banana. Another technique for enlivening a mess night was for someone to suddenly turn out the lights and ignite a thunder flash, stuff it into a bag of flour and hurl it into the room. The result was a blinding flash, a large bang, a smell reminiscent of freshly baked bread and a resultant even-coating of flour over everyone, visible when the lights came back on.

Whilst on exercise in Germany, the fact that I was a geriatrician came to the notice of one of the senior officers, who was involved in the guarding of Rudolph Hess, in Spandau Prison, in West Berlin. Hess had been unwell and the authorities were considering getting a specialist opinion. They thought I might fit the bill. Although I had no actual involvement, one of the regular medics sidled up to me and warned me that there could be problems.

He had examined Rudolph Hess some years before. Rudolph Hess was in fact a friend of Hitler's and effectively, his deputy. They had served together in WW1 and the medical records of Rudolph Hess bore testament to gunshot wounds which he had sustained to the shoulder which had left scarring. It was claimed that the man in Spandau, who had been imprisoned since 1947, had no such evidence of gunshot wounds on his body. This has led to a conspiracy theory that the man in

Spandau was not Hess. It has been publicised and theorised that the original Rudolph Hess died in 1941, possibly at the hands of the SS, who were jealous of his relationship with Hitler and it was a substitute who flew to Scotland in 1941 to attempt peace talks. In support of the theory it has been noted that for twenty-eight years following his imprisonment in Spandau, Hess refused to see his family in person. His death in 1987 has been claimed to have been due to suicide by hanging but it is also claimed that his arthritis would have precluded self-harm. The cable with which he was hanged was destroyed and the shed where it happened burned down very shortly afterwards.

A very interesting survival weekend exercise was conducted, courtesy of the SAS. I stress that this was a weekend exercise and limited. Nonetheless, some techniques learned have remained with me:

• To get through a barbed wire fence safely and by leaving little trace, is remarkably easy. Do not try to climb over, go through it. There is normally enough give in such fences for someone to put a boot on the bottom two wires, to produce a gap and then pull up the top two strands, to reveal a sufficiently wide gap to step through. It is obviously easier if you have an accomplice.

• Protection from the elements and camouflage may be needed temporarily or for longer periods. Y-shaped poles, cut from a tree and embedded into the soil, can be used to support ridge poles across the top of the 'Y'. Smaller poles propped up and then secured with twine, provide the sides, with twigs tied across that, providing a base for some thatching. Basic temporary thatch can be created by turf or autumn leaves thrown upon it from the base, upwards.

- Water can be obtained from digging a gypsy well. The technique is fairly simple. It involves digging a hole of about eight inches deep in damp ground. That hole will gradually fill with muddy water. That water should be bailed out and the next refill ought to be much clearer. The final filtration process can be achieved using a plastic soft drinks bottle, with the base cut off. Pack the neck end with some sphagnum moss, followed by a thick layer of peat or charcoal, topped again with sphagnum moss. If the water is then poured through that mixture, it ought to be relatively safe to drink.

- There are some unconventional ways of making fire. Soaking dried tinder with antifreeze and adding potassium permanganate will cause spontaneous combustion. Sparking an ordinary battery with wire wool will cause it to glow and will become sufficiently hot to ignite dry tinder.

- Worms can be dug up and fried, providing a source of protein. Most plants, even if edible, have little food value and there is no guarantee that because birds, mammals or insects eat a plant that it is safe for human consumption. There are some standard techniques to minimise risk with strange plants. Firstly, check that the plant is in good condition and neither slimy nor wormy. Leaves which when crushed smell of bitter almonds or peaches, are probably poisonous. Rub or squeeze some of the juice of the plant on a tender part of the body and discard any plant that causes discomfort, rash or swelling. Try the juice on the lips, in the corner of the mouth, on the tip of the tongue and under the tongue and then chew. If there is any soreness, irritation, stinging, or burning, discard. The next step is to swallow a small amount and wait a minimum of six hours, to test reaction. As a general rule, avoid any plants with a milky sap. Avoid plants that are red. Avoid fruit, which is divided into five segments.

Bomb disposal lectures are usually both entertaining and informative. The lecture room, which I attended on one occasion, had been pre-stocked with various timing devices to produce explosions at random throughout the lecture. Makeshift incendiary devices can be created by tucking a lit cigarette into a book of matches. The 'fuse' can be adjusted by the distance between the lit end and the match heads. The humble Christmas party popper can be used as a distraction. Simply, remove the streamers and replace with a grape. Anchor it appropriately, such that when a door or drawer is opened, the party popper is set off, causing an explosion. This will obviously not be lethal but can be a useful distraction if necessary.

Joining the TA is relatively straightforward for basic recruits but more complex for those wishing a commission. Commissioned officers have to sign the Official Secrets Act and before a commission is granted, they are security screened. Family screening routinely goes back for three generations and just occasionally, dark secrets are revealed. I know of one person denied a commission in the TA when it was revealed that his great uncle had been imprisoned for crimes against the state. He had had a major role in the IRA, following the Easter rising of 1916. Another potentially promising officer had this aspect of his career ruined when it was revealed that his grandfather had been a communist, involved in the miner's strike in 1926. Soldiers, and in particular officers, need to be physically fit. The least blemish on a medical record is sufficient for rejection. Asthma is characterised by attacks of severe breathlessness and wheezing. Any such soldier with an attack is not only incapacitated himself but may take out from combat one or two other able bodied soldiers to assist him to a treatment centre. The smoke and potential gas on a battle field can produce such attacks. Therefore, the least hint of asthma in medical records is cause for rejection. This unfortunately can catch out those who have no real asthma but were labelled as such by well-meaning doctors. The usual circumstances were that someone, aged 13ish, disliked organised games at school and tried to wriggle out of them. By feigning a little bit of wheeziness, they were able to acquire a doctor's note, excusing them from future games. This has come back to haunt many people.

Potential officers undergo quite strenuous training, which can involve shortages of food and drink coupled with sleep deprivation. One such one potential officer fainted, probably due to a combination of tiredness and lack of food, but was seen to twitch (fainting is often associated with some twitching, due to the brain being temporarily hypoxic). This is not epilepsy. However, if twitching is witnessed, it is often labelled as epilepsy and very difficult to have this removed from medical records. For the same reasons, as with asthma, epilepsy is an absolute contraindication to recruitment, on the basis that an epileptic fit can incapacitate not only the victim but also those who are required to provide assistance.

Successful recruits into the TA are invariably extroverts. They would often be keen and bright and enthusiastic. These are clearly the traits required of an efficient soldier. Towards the end of WW1, the German officer cadre was running out of enthusiastic bright young men. The categories left were the bright but idle, the keen but stupid and the stupid and idle. The bright but idle and the stupid and idle were not particularly desirable reservoirs from which to recruit. However, the stupid and enthusiastic were to be avoided at all costs, simply because they would pursue their stupid ideas with great enthusiasm. TA recruits came from all walks of life, bringing diverse skills. Some skills, frowned upon in civilised society, can be extremely useful at times of adversity. I learnt how to hotwire a car and to use a tennis ball to circumvent central locking mechanisms on cars of the vintage available in the 1980s. The technique was simple. Cut a small circular hole, the size of a ten pence piece, in the tennis ball, which is then placed over the driver's lock. By punching the tennis ball hard, a significant amount of air is introduced into the locking mechanism, with the pleasing result of seeing all the doors unlock. One older sergeant had been a child during the exceptional hard winter of 1947. Matters were made worse by fuel shortages. Their back garden backed onto a busy railway line. His father had set up a garishly painted makeshift coconut shy in the back garden, close to the railway line. The result was an abundance of coal. The young railway firemen could not resist the temptation and almost all the firemen would throw chunks of coal to try to dislodge the coconuts.

Exposure to cold has long been considered an important factor in causing respiratory diseases. Even though we know that respiratory infections are viral or bacterial, it is still a general belief amongst clinicians that the chilling of the body exerts a predisposing influence to such infections. In fact, this is not borne out by experimental evidence. Self-experimentation was conducted in America in 1916. One brave fifty-seven-year-old doctor, prone to catarrh and frequent attacks of bronchitis, subjected himself to some twenty-seven separate experiments to detect the potential adverse effects on exposure to severe cold. After hot baths, after ice cold baths and even when suffering from an acute cold, he exposed himself naked to cold air and drafts at temperatures well below 10°c and sometimes below 0° for periods varying from twenty minutes to one hour. Such exposure often caused severe shaking chills but there were no permanent effects of any kind and no symptoms of any of the pathological conditions, usually ascribed to exposure to cold.

The army requires some in-house skills, only at time of war and almost never during times of peace. In times of peace, laundries are not provided by the military themselves nor are railway services. All these can be out-sourced. However, in the event of the breakdown of normal peaceful activities, such skills become vital. There are specialised TA railway units, which draw on professional civilian skills to provide the army with the manpower and experience in time of war. There were also laundry platoons, which were originally formed in response to the needs of the western desert campaigns of WW2, where there were no laundries to be commandeered. Laundry platoons used to often train with general hospital units, in preparation for their potential combat roles. One such platoon had been provided with robust heavy duty kit, which had been captured from the Germans in the 1940s. It was in perfect working order. In essence, a laundry platoon ought to be able to wash, dry and iron the kit of six hundred men within a few hours and also provide them with showers.

One of the catholic padres gave us an illustrated talk about the crypt of the Capuchins in Rome. In 1631, the Capuchin friars left their friary in Rome, near the Trevi fountain, and relocated in what were the then suburbs. This has now been subsumed by greater Rome and lies within walking distance of the central railway station. When they relocated, they took the remains of the deceased friars with them. Legend has it that when they moved, they brought three hundred cart loads of their deceased friars and interned them in the burial crypt under the present church with soil brought from Jerusalem. Gradually, over the years, a vast number of bones were used to create six crypts, which are generally considered to be works of art. The crypt of the resurrection is created from various parts of the human skeleton to form a frame for the picture of Jesus commanding Lazarus to come out alive from the tomb. There are human bones everywhere, with large numbers being nailed to the walls in intricate patterns. Many are piled high upon others, whilst others again hang from the ceiling as light fixtures. Though once described as 'the most horrifying images in all of Christendom' it is not supposed to be a macabre display but a silent reminder of the quick passage of life on earth and the mortality of human beings. As monks died during the lifetime of the crypt, the longest buried monk was exhumed to make room for the newly deceased, who were buried without coffins. The newly reclaimed bones were added to the decorative motifs. I subsequently visited this crypt and would recommend it for anyone who is in Rome.

He also had a vast repertoire of anecdotes, which had appeared in church bulletins or were announced in services, some of which were:

• Bertha Belch, a missionary from Africa, will be speaking tonight in the church hall. Come along and hear Bertha Belch all the way from Africa.

- We announce a national prayer and fasting conference. The cost for attending the fasting and prayer conference includes meals.

- Miss Mary Jones sang 'I will not pass this way again', giving obvious pleasure to the congregation.

- Ladies, do not forget the rummage sale, it is a chance to get rid of those things not worth keeping around the house. Don't forget to bring your husbands.

- The peacekeeping meeting scheduled for today has been cancelled at short notice, due to a conflict. This morning's service will be 'Jesus walks on the water', with the sermon tonight being entitled 'Searching for Jesus'.

- Father Murphy will give his farewell message after which there will be singing of 'break forth into joy'.

- Don't let worry kill you off – let the church help.

- John Smith and Jenny Carter were married on October the 24th, in church. So ends a friendship that began in their school days.

- At the evening service, the sermon topic will be 'What is hell'? Come early and listen to our choir practice.

- In honour of Easter Sunday, Mrs Johnson will come forward and lay an egg on the altar.

- Weight watchers will meet at 7.00 pm in the church hall. Please use the large double doors at the side entrance.

- The low self-esteem support group will meet on Thursdays at 7.00 pm. Please use the back door.

- The ladies of the church have castoff clothing of every kind. They may be seen in the basement on Friday afternoon.

- For those of you who have children and don't know it, we have a nursery downstairs.

I heard of a man who had attended a conference in Northern Ireland, during the marching season. He and his wife had been standing in the crowd in a small town, when the men in bowler hats marched solidly by. His wife enquired as to who was this 'King Billy' they keep talking about? The response from a large woman in front was that she ought to go away and read her bible. Apparently, carrots were originally purple but were genetically modified to their current orange colour as a tribute to William of Orange.

Once upon a time, there was a non-conformist swallow, who decided not to fly south for the winter. However, soon the winter turned so cold that he was reluctantly forced to go. In a short period, ice formed on his wings and he fell to earth in a farmyard, almost frozen. A cow passed by and crapped on the little swallow. The swallow thought it was the end, but the manure warmed him and defrosted his wings. Warm and happy and able to breathe, he started to sing. Just then, a large cat came by and hearing the chirping, investigated the sounds. The cat cleared away the manure, found the chirping bird and promptly ate him. Now, there are four morals to this story:

- Everyone who shits on you is not necessarily your enemy.

• Everyone who gets you out of the shit is not necessarily your friend.

• If you are warm and happy in a pile of shit, keep your mouth shut.

• If it smells bad, it probably is.

One of the great slogans of military life is 'Train hard, fight easy' – as true today as when first stated. Another lesson is that persecution of enemies serves only to strengthen their resolve and any martyrdom which results serves only to be an effective recruiting sergeant. Of the two forces in the world, never in the history of warfare has the sword overpowered the spirit. This has been true of many conflicts but perhaps best illustrated by the lengthy conflicts in Vietnam, which started soon after the French tried to reclaim Indochina, after the defeat of the Japanese, who had occupied the country. The Vietnamese guerrillas, known as the Viet Minh and commanded by General Giap, waged guerrilla warfare. By February 1954, the French forces had chosen to force a decisive battle with them at Dien Bien Phu. The idea was to draw the guerrillas into a major confrontation that would cripple them. They manned it with many of their best soldiers, the paratroopers and the French foreign legionnaires, who prepared an extensive system of fortifications, supplied by an airfield. Dien Bien Phu was set deep in the hills of northwest Vietnam and positioned so as to cut off Viet Minh supply lines from the neighbouring kingdom of Laos, However, General Giap surrounded them and besieged the French. The Viet Minh had large numbers of heavy artillery, which they dismantled and carried up the mountain and then reassembled them on the hillsides, such as to overlook the whole French encampment. Following tenacious fighting on the ground and persistent bombardment, the French positions were overrun and their perimeter contracted, such as to deprive the French of air supply. A two month siege ended in French surrender. The French eventually withdraw all of their forces from colonies in French Indochina but stipulated that Vietnam would be temporarily divided at the seventeenth parallel, with control of the north given to the Viet Minh, led by Ho Chi Minh, and the south becoming the State of Vietnam, nominally under the control of the Emperor. This effectively prevented Ho Chi Minh gaining control of the entire country. The refusal to allow elections in 1956, as had been stipulated by the Peace Accord, eventually set the scene for the involvement of the US, with military forces on the ground, and the rest is history.

The will to fight and the resourcefulness of the Vietnamese, has to be admired. Supplies to the Vietcong in the south were brought down the Ho Chi Minh trail, running down the western border of Vietnam, mostly carried on the backs of volunteers. Vietcong bases in the south were strategically placed and were mostly underground. The American air base at Da Nang was overlooked by Marble Mountain and caves therein provided cover for hidden artillery periodically hauled up by hand and used with devastating short term effect before the Vietcong escaped. The Cu Chi tunnels, just outside of Saigon, were a permanent base and are now a major tourist attraction. That area is mostly a sandstone hillock in a bend of the river, with a complex of tunnels, three stories deep, tunnelled in by hand. There was a sophisticated ventilation system, with the air vents on the surface cleverly disguised as termite hills. Even though the tunnels have been widened slightly for the benefit of tourists, they are a very tight squeeze, even for a scantily clad adult male of European origin. They would have been almost impossible to negotiate by U S soldiers carrying equipment. Entrances were well disguised by small trap doors and the top layer was in part protected from high explosive bombs by bits of captured American tanks being used to reinforce the ceilings. To prevent American access, the tunnels were heavily protected with various forms of pit traps and spikes. At the intersection in tunnels, there would often be three passages. One went on into the depths; another led down to the river as an escape route and a third was a progressively narrowing tunnel which led nowhere. The complexes were well supplied with large chambers deep underground providing medical facilities, sleeping accommodation and kitchens. The smoke from the kitchens was led out along large bamboo pipes, to be released slowly into bushes, up to a hundred yards from the hidden bases.

When the Americans bombed Hanoi and Haiphong harbour, they were aware that the Vietnamese had surface-to-air missiles supplied to them by the Russians, and mounted their attacks above the ceiling range of these missiles. Unbeknown to them, the Vietnamese had managed to increase the effective height of these missiles, and caused some devastating damage to the B52 bombers. The famous Ho Chi Minh sandal, a flip flop made from car tyres, was cleverly designed to leave the foot prints as the opposite, such that footprints seemingly going from south to north were in fact made by people travelling north to south.

After a mess dinner, the tale was related of a visit to a variety show in a city, where the high spot of the evening was a striptease by a buxom blonde. At the climax of her act, the lady removed the last of her clothing, behind a screen, which was in fact a flock of white doves, perched on a stand. A soldier in the front row, frustrated at being denied a glimpse of her in her 'all together', drew a pistol and fired off a blank cartridge. The exposed performer stood open-mouthed in shock for a few moments, before rushing off stage. The doves meanwhile fluttered around the theatre, depositing evidence of their displeasure, on the heads of the audience.

Army issue toilet paper was of the shiny, medicated tracing-paper variety and universally known as "John Wayne paper". It took shit off no-one!

Fritz Darges, was a Waffen-SS officer, appointed as an adjutant to Hitler in January 1944. During a strategic conference in the following July, a fly apparently landed on Hitler's shoulder. He ordered Darges to kill it. Darges suggested that as it was an airborne pest, the job should go to the Luftwaffe adjutant. Hitler lost his temper, fired him on the spot and had him banished to the eastern front.

There are only thirty villages in England which have been deemed 'thankful' villages. They are distinguished by having no war memorials, because all those who served in world war one came home safely.

Contrary to rumour R.A.M.C does not stand for "Robbed all my comrades." Also, the officer cadre of the illustrious Cheshire Regiment are not described as the "Cream of the British Army" because they are rich, thick and full of clots.

CHAPTER ELEVEN

Management

"Big fleas have little fleas upon their backs to bite them. Little fleas have lesser fleas and so on ad infinitum" – such is the world.

The NHS came into being at a time of national austerity, whilst rationing was still in force. It was a service, and that ethos of service from people who had left the military services continued. There was a 'make do and mend' mentality and patients were generally undemanding and grateful. Waiting lists were an acceptable feature, which allowed supply to dictate demand. The ultimate gatekeeper was the general practitioner, who limited hospital referrals. The facilities, which the NHS inherited, included the old voluntary hospitals, the municipal hospitals and the poor law institutions. Decommissioned military hospitals built for the Canadian and US armies, provided additional resource and were also taken over by the NHS.

The management was top down with the Minister of Health being ultimately responsible. There was a general assumption that once the backlog of disease had been dealt with, NHS expenditure would plateau and then decrease as the population became healthier. Hospitals were primarily designed for the needs of single illness and the concept of multiple co-morbidity was alien to most, apart from a handful of budding geriatricians. By the mid-1970s, management of the NHS had become structured by yet another reorganisation. There were regional Health Authorities, which determined strategy. These were subdivided into Area Health Authorities, which provided the local administration. The districts provided the day-to-day hospital care, usually set around the structure of a district general hospital. These were the hubs of the NHS. As a general rule, each had a casualty department, serviced by medical, surgical, orthopaedic and often a paediatric ward. Actual bed numbers depended upon the size of the district. Maternity services were often located within district general hospitals but sometimes historic reasons dictated that they were located offsite, elsewhere and sometimes co-located with long stay geriatric wards – "Hatch and dispatch units". A hospital bed is not just a "bed"; it is a unit of hospital resource which includes the entire infrastructure to support the level of illness of the patient therein. Without that backup, which will include enough very skilled staff, equipment etc. the bed is effectively useless. Very seriously ill patients require greater backup. This backup is a finite resource. On that basis, beds cannot be made available at short notice merely by dint of human endeavour.

Funding of beds was dictated by the population. Specialised units were normally centrally funded by the region and locations varied. The Mersey Region had chosen to distribute regional centres, so as to provide district general hospitals with their own highly specialised units, of which to be proud. Whiston Hospital had the Burns Unit, Walton Hospital had the Neurological Unit and Clatterbridge Hospital had the Cancer Regional Centre. Broadgreen Hospital continued to provide the Regional Heart and Chest Unit.

Because the funding was dependent upon population, Liverpool Area Health Authority had a major funding problem owing to the population falling during the 70's and 80's. Slum clearance had relocated people to Kirkby and Skelmersdale and the economic downturn caused many young families to leave in search of work and better prospects. The population left was ageing. Liverpool was "over churched", "over schooled", "over pubbed" and had too many hospital beds. Funding problems were aggravated by Broadgreen Hospital being at the extreme eastern periphery of the health authority boundary. You could literally throw a tennis ball from Broadgreen's grounds into the neighbouring territory of Knowsley and St Helens, whose designated DGH, Whiston Hospital, was 5 miles away. Thus, for some 2 miles to the east of Broadgreen Hospital, this local population of some 50,000 people in the "Whiston bulge" or "Huyton salient", preferentially looked to Broadgeen to provide elective and emergency medical services, even though Whiston Hospital was actually receiving the funding. Ambulances responding to 999 calls from this area also brought emergencies to A&E.

The day-to-day management within the hospital was normally run by a senior consultant, matron and the hospital administrator. Various committees assisted and much power was held by the medical board, comprised of the hospital consultants. Doctors were generally involved in the simple administration and day-to-day tasks, rather than strategic management, unless they were public health doctors based at headquarters.

Back in the 1980s, and in response to an advert placed in the British Medical Journal for a Locum SHO in geriatric medicine for Newsham General Hospital, a Dr G applied for the post. He had submitted a handwritten letter and CV in support of his application. His contact details were care of a hospital in the southwest of England and a phone number provided. He appeared to 'tick' all the boxes and I made contact with him, on at least three occasions, by phone. On each occasion, I got through to the Hospital switchboard, who connected me to the extension provided, which happened to be the ward phone. It was normally answered by one of the nurses, who alerted Dr G, who then came to the phone. We went through his CV and he gave me a satisfactory explanation for some of the more unusual elements within. In particular, he explained that he had given up a principal post in general practice upon a change in domestic circumstances, in order to pursue his original desire of a career in hospital medicine. Normally, he would have been invited to a formal interview before commencing work. However, this would have involved him in at least a three hundred mile trip, for what in essence was a two week locum post. I was able to obtain good references over the phone from the secretaries of two consultants, whilst the third referee was away on leave and no reference was on file. On the strength of these references and upon the impression he gave over the phone, I contacted him again and suggested that he should present himself to me, on Monday morning, for a short informal interview, in anticipation of him commencing work later that day. I informed him of the statutory need for him to have pre-employment health screening and the need to present his usual credentials to the appropriate personnel officer. The personnel department arranged for single accommodation to be available for him on site, in anticipation of his arrival, at some point at his convenience, during the preceding weekend.

On the designated Monday, he presented himself to me at shortly after 11.30 am. I had tried to chase him up earlier but received some excuses. When I met with him, at 11.30 am, his appearance at that time caused me considerable alarm. He was unsteady on his feet, had slurring of speech and smelled strongly of alcohol. I formed the not unreasonable opinion that he was extremely drunk and requested an explanation. His excuse was that he had arrived late the night before, whereupon he had received bad news concerning the sudden death of an estranged child from a previous marriage. He had drowned his sorrows. It was quite apparent that he was unfit to be interviewed and I sent him away to his room, agreeing to reappraise the situation the following day, when he was sober. The following day, and although he was yet to be officially appointed, he had collected a bleep and had gone onto a ward. The ward sister, upon smelling alcohol again on his breath, fortunately had the common sense to confine him to the ward office. Upon my arrival on that ward, shortly after 9 am, it was quite apparent that he was drunk again. I escorted him for a walk around the grounds, where we had the opportunity to talk. He admitted to having a problem with alcohol and on the basis that he was ill, I sent him back to his room and promised to arrange some medical follow up. I was later somewhat embarrassed to discover the following:

- That his place of residence for the six weeks prior to my meeting him was as an inpatient in a psychiatric ward, where he was 'drying out.'

- The telephone conversations that we had with him were when he was an inpatient, not working on the ward, as I had supposed.

- He was discharged from the psychiatric unit in anticipation that he was cured and had a job.

- He had actually arrived at Newsham Hospital on the Friday night, not the Sunday evening, as he had told me. His first port of call had been to the pub opposite, where he had established his credentials with the landlord and obtained a crate of whiskey 'on tick'. He had spent the whole weekend being extremely drunk and other resident doctors and some of the porters had been involved, on a number of occasions, in retrieving him from an unconscious state in the grounds and escorting him back to his room

It further transpired that he had a formidable reputation for inebriation on duty and had been dismissed from a number of posts in the southwest for repeated drunken incapacity. He was however now ensconced in a room at Newsham Hospital. He had never technically started work but clearly needed some sort of help. In order for him to have a psychiatric referral, he needed a general practitioner. One of the local general practitioners agreed to take him on his books, as a temporary resident and made a provisional appointment for him to be seen early on the following Friday's evening surgery. Dr G duly appeared, again obviously drunk. He introduced himself as Dr G to the receptionist, in a loud slurred voice. The packed waiting room formed the impression that he was coming as that evening's locum doctor and to-a-man, they disappeared. The GP had seen his last patient by 5.30pm. Dr G was eventually admitted to the local psychiatric unit, for another attempt at drying him out. Unfortunately, when he arrived at Newsham, he had brought in tow, his girlfriend, a young Irish girl of about seventeen years of age. She herself was pleasant enough but somewhat innocent. When I asked whether she was concerned about his heavy drinking, she offered the observation that compared to the men in her family; she thought his drinking was relatively moderate. It took some six weeks before she finally left the premises.

Although I could defend each and every step I had taken on this painful journey, the District Medical Officer, who was technically my boss, remained po-faced and was clearly not amused.

By the late 1980s, Newsham General Hospital had closed and the patients had been relocated to newly built accommodation at Broadgreen Hospital. This was marvellous. We were now on the site of a DGH, with the support of other physicians, specialist medical units, surgery and I could receive acutely ill patients through the A&E. However, within some twelve months, matters were to unravel. The great and the good had conducted a pan-Liverpool review on the future provision of services. This was more about the saving of money than the actual provision of services. Amongst other rationalisations, the big money saver was to close the A&E department on the Broadgreen site. This would turn off instantly the flow of unfunded patients from the "Huyton salient", forcing them to use their designated district general hospital. Furthermore, once the hospital ceased to receive unselected acutely ill patients, all the expensive support facilities could gradually be cut back. There would be no need for a blood bank around the clock, there would be no need for an x-ray department around the clock, and there would be no need for operating theatres to be available around the clock. Slowly but surely, all this came to pass and there was a general transfer of all acute services from the Broadgreen site, to the Royal Liverpool Hospital and on occasions, elsewhere. It was poorly planned. Everything had the smack of services finding their own level in the absence of support facilities, rather than there being any strategic or operational plan. With the operating theatres being closed in the evenings, most acute surgeons decamped. As a consequence, there were patients who developed surgical complications on the Broadgreen site, who failed to receive timely surgical opinion or operation.

Achieving Trust Status was seen by staff as a means of resisting the closure of A&E. NHS Trusts came into existence in 1991. They have now been in existence for more than twenty-five years and most NHS staff have not worked under any other form of management. Various reorganisations have continued.

"We trained very hard, but it seemed that every time we were beginning to form into teams, we would be reorganised. I was to learn later in life that we tend to meet any new situation by reorganising – and a wonderful method it can be for creating the illusion of progress, whilst producing confusion, inefficiency and demoralisation". This quote, which has adorned many the wall of hospital consultants, is normally attributed to Gaius Petronius, a Roman Consul. It was however more likely crafted by a disgruntled WW2 officer and posted on a notice board in a transit camp.

Broadgreen Hospital staff embraced with great enthusiasm, the concept of Trust status. Money was now supposed to follow patients and the senior staff believed that if they continued to provide a good service, the patients would continue to come and that would include those from the "Huyton salient". If money followed patients, then suddenly Broadgreen would receive a considerable increase in funding and the future of the hospital, including A&E, would be assured. However, this was predicated on the naive presumption that all would be left to the free-market. In fact, the money did not follow patients and purchasers chose not to buy the services, which we had provided. Unfortunately, Broadgreen had invested heavily in infrastructure and staff and lack of purchase of services led to technical "bankruptcy" which precipitated merger with the Royal.

When Trusts became Trusts, suddenly the day-to-day management of that which had previously been organised by the Area Health Authority, devolved to the individual hospitals. The phones were to be funded direct from hospital monies, as were the rates and the usual utility bills, including water, gas and electricity. Not all managers were up to the challenges.

The Peter Principle was first observed by Dr Laurence J. Peter and published in his book "The Peter Principle" in 1968. This was an observation that in an organizational hierarchy, every employee will rise or get promoted to his or her level of incompetence. It is based on the notion that employees will get promoted as long as they are competent but at some point, will fail to get promoted beyond a certain job because it has become too challenging for them. Employees thus rise to their level of incompetence and stay there. Over time, every position in the hierarchy will be filled by someone who is not competent enough to carry out his or her new duties. Promotion to the higher-ranking posts may not necessarily reveal the employee's incompetence if the job stays the same as it was on appointment. However, most job content changes and the new position may require different skills the employee does not possess or cannot learn. Dr Peter summed up matters with the saying: "the cream rises until it sours." This is a big problem in the NHS. Perfectly competent clinical staff, often senior ward managers (sisters/charge nurses), are tempted away from the bedside into management roles initially well within their competence. All is well until the job changes such as to require competency in something in which they have neither skill nor interest, by which time they may have been clinically de-skilled. Many become uneasy, unhappy, stressed and some take early retirement. Theoretically this can be solved through continued education. However even with proper employee training, the Peter Principle predicts the employee will eventually get to a position where they are incompetent because of further promotion.

This story was doing the rounds a few years ago:-

A woman in a hot air balloon realised she was lost. She descended a bit more and shouted, "Excuse me can you help me? I promised a friend I would meet him an hour ago, but I don't know where I am."

The man below replied, "You're in a hot air balloon hovering approximately 10 metres above the ground at grid reference 98/58."

"You're very precise, are you a doctor?" said the balloonist.

"I am," replied the man, "how did you know?"

"Well," answered the balloonist, "everything you've told me is probably technically correct, but I've no idea what to make of the information and the fact is I'm still lost. Frankly, you've not been much help at all. If anything, you've delayed my trip by our talk."

The man below responded, "You must be in NHS management."

"I am," replied the balloonist, "but how did you know?"

"Well," said the man, "you don't know where you are or where you're going. You have risen to where you are due to a large quantity of hot air. You made a promise which you have no idea how to keep, and you expect people like me beneath you to solve your problems. The fact is that you are in exactly the same position you were before we met, but now, somehow, it's my fault."

Spasticity is a medical term for muscle rigidity and paresis means weakness/mild paralysis. Spastic paresis is common after stroke. Many years ago, a prestigious neurological unit doing research on spastic paresis e-mailed UK physicians requesting help with their study. The response was minimal! The word "spastic" was politically incorrect and the e-mail was blocked by the filters. Sadly, proper medical words of yesteryear such as moron, idiot, imbecile and cretin which one can see written in very old records now convey different connotations.

The Dunning-Kruger effect, named after David Dunning and Justin Kruger of Cornell University, occurs when people fail to adequately assess their level of competence – or more importantly, their incompetence – at a task and thus consider themselves much more competent than everyone else. This lack of awareness/insight is attributed to their lower level of competence robbing them of the ability to critically analyse their performance, leading to a significant overestimate of themselves. The inverse also applies: competent people tend to underestimate their ability compared to others.

During one summer, shortly after it achieved trust status, Broadgreen came up with an innovative scheme to save on the cost of water. A "nodding donkey" drill appeared on site and underwent test drilling around the site. It looked like Texas had come to Knotty Ash. In due course an artesian aquifer was tapped into adjacent to the detached self-contained mortuary! This was a geologic layer of porous and permeable sand and gravel, through which water flowed and was stored. An artesian aquifer is normally confined between impermeable rocks or clay and has positive pressure. The well-head was connected to the hospital reservoir and mains water disconnected. Now whilst the water was potable, it tasted horrible. Most staff would come to work bearing litres of their own domestic tap-water for beverages. Around this time there was subsidence on site, mostly confined to those single storey structures which had been erected during the War as emergency wards. They were no longer in use as wards but provided space for ancillary services and offices. They had to be shored up at great expense. Whether the subsidence was related to the tapping of the well or not, I don't know, though the well was quietly capped and use of mains water resumed.

New EU regulations rendered the on-site Hospital incinerator obsolete. Rather than bear the expense of sending waste elsewhere a new incinerator was purchased and the building to house it constructed. On the day it was "sparked up" for the first time, clinical waste was loaded into it. The following day the local paper contained the headline "Black smuts fall over Knotty Ash". There was some fundamental problem with it and I don't think it was ever used again.

I took on the role as Clinical Director. Doctors in general are highly educated but can be mavericks. They like to be in charge and dislike taking orders from intellectual inferiors. They can be easily tempted to take positions of power! From management perspective, they would rather have doctors "inside the tent, pissing out, rather than outside, causing trouble by pissing in". Doctors were being encouraged to take on management roles even though formal training was absent and support minimal. This is where TA experience held me in good stead. I pass on my advice. Firstly source 4 filing cabinets for use as follows:-

• Label the first with "P" – this is for any letter referring to any action described as a priority – there will be many.

• Label the second "PLUS" – this is for any letter demanding a positive action.

• Label the third "MINUS" – this is for any letter demanding a negative reaction.

• Label the fourth "M" – this is for minutes of meetings.

You will now rapidly collect the vital tools to respond to any situation. Cross referencing the Plus and Minus files will give you the ammunition to choose whether to act positively or negatively to any instruction. Priorities, by definition, take precedence and you can only have one priority at a time – you choose. The minutes file will prove the futility of meetings. When the minutes of a previous medical board meeting were read out and approved as an accurate record of that meeting a month earlier, they turned out to be those of three years before – nothing had changed! More on meetings later.

At my expense I obtained education on management practice from Boston USA, not exactly Harvard but from the ultimate (top secret) source which I cannot divulge. The essentials of keeping management control are:-

- Create a slogan (the word means a Scottish Highlander war cry) to inspire. Good slogans include "total quality management", "achieving excellence", "complaints are jewels to be savoured not duels to be fought", "It's a new paradigm" and "it's an opportunity not a problem".

- Pretend to care – learn to hear without listening.

- Incentivise. Introduce an employee of the month award, tell people that no-one else can do what they can do as well as them and that they are valued members of the team.

- Keep staff too busy to cause dissent. Task trouble-makers with organising team-work exercises, writing mission statements, preparing status reports and preparing lists of potential new names for the department.

- Re-organise or at least threaten to do so frequently.

- Avoid making actual management decisions yourself – not much good comes from most management decisions and you need deniability. This can be achieved by forming a task force of people too busy to meet, requesting more data and loosing key documents. Form a committee to make the decision.

- When something so bad needs to be done and you fear leaving your DNA on the scene get "Human resources" involved.

- Form teams. Although a team is more like a convoy than a committee all move at the speed of the slowest. By randomly inserting or removing someone intellectually challenged, a skilled manager can easily control speed of progress.

Doctors are generally bad team players; they often have leadership skills but few have "followership skills". When leading, they give orders on the basis that they are running a benevolent dictatorship not a democracy. When they are mere members they have a tendency to go "off message" and do their own thing – handling this as a manager is tricky. The standard ploy is to embarrass the maverick in front of the team with the phrase "There is no "I" in team". However so much medical training has involved public bollockings that most Consultants are immune. One such individual approaching retirement responded to that phrase used by a bossy nurse manager with the riposte "I agree but there is a "U" in c*nt" before storming off.

Educational meetings are the medical professions preferred means of having fun, gaining "CPD" points and showing off their skills and intellect. Two or three day conferences on paid study leave are the epitome. Historically these were heavily subsidised by pharmaceutical companies promoting their products. Although I knew of few whose prescribing was skewed by lavish hospitality it is now heavily regulated and virtually non-existent nowadays. Many years ago on the first of April, I was sent an invitation to a conference in a posh hotel. The details as I recollect were:-

UPDATE IN PERINEAL HYGIENE TECHNIQUES

0900 Arrival & Registration

09.15 Chairman's introduction – Prof Phil McCavity – Belfast, will invite contributions.

09.30 Post-menopausal problems – Dr Fanny Smellie – Edinburgh.

10.00 Anatomy/physiology of defaecation – Prof Hugh Janus – Cardiff.

10.30 Coffee and chocolate brownies.

11.00 Anal wiping – a cultural perspective from the Middle East focussing on the problems associated with left hand amputation by explosives.

11.30 Prof Leck Meinarsch (Vienna) gives a European perspective focussing upon his shocking research findings of arse-wiping denial in rural Austria.

12.00 Sister Melina Heaps, from Scunthorpe Hospitals Intermediate Trust, describes the use of the Bristol Stool Chart and the job satisfaction of working daily in S.H.I.T.

12.30 Lunch sponsored by "Sniff & Phew".

13.30 Prof Crapper describes the world before the flushable WC – the history of the use of grass, bracken, sponges and paper.

14.30 Dr Wiap Mi Ass (Shanghai) gives a Far East perspective and will describe techniques of maintaining hygiene during the Shi-Ting dynasty.

15.00 Drs Ben Dover and Wiap Mi Ass discuss paediatric techniques to maintain anal cleanliness.

15.30 Prof Ivor Procter-Scope will lead the practical session and small group work – please volunteer.

16.00 Tea and sponge.

16.30 Plenary session – led by Dr Emma Royd will be a "gloves off" question and answer session – blood may be let.

18.00 Cocktails sponsored by "Bottoms Up".

19.00 Conference dinner.

CHAPTER TWELVE

More on Management

In my capacity as Clinical Director, I received a letter from management seeking help in making a claim for reimbursement of excess council rates previously paid. The basis was that they had statistics which suggested there had been long stay patients (60 days and over) in our unit – long stay patients apparently exempt their facilities from having to pay rates. I looked back through my records for the relevant year. It had been a busy but gratifying year. In accordance with the desires of the new NHS Trust to maximise patient throughput, we had laboured long and hard. Our acute geriatric unit, with ninety-six beds, had admitted a record 3,500 patients during that year. Standards had been maintained, even though it had been necessary to outlie patients in surgical wards, when demand exceeded supply. The official statistics supplied by the region freely acknowledged our record throughput. Bed occupancy was noted at 105% but we received criticism for having the worst performance in the region, with an average length of stay amounting to forty days with some lengths of stay being recorded as in excess of sixty days.

This was clearly wrong and I pointed out that a simple' back of the envelope' calculation would suggest that if 3,500 patients passed through 100 beds a year, then some 35 patients would occupy each bed per annum. It was a simple step to divide the figure of 35 into 365 days of the year, in order to obtain a figure for average length of stay of just over 10 days. That would have made us one of the most efficient units in the region. Alternatively, if 3,500 patients had indeed stayed an average of forty days, we would have required 100% occupancy of almost 400 beds continually, during the year. The data were clearly incongruous but officialdom continued to support those regional statistics, resulting in the letter which I had received. It took some years for common sense to prevail. What had happened? Quite simply, it was discovered that for two patients, their date of birth had been erroneously recorded as the date of admission. Two octogenarians had been officially logged as each having spent some 80 years as inpatients. Fortunately, this produced such a gross skewing of the statistics that it was eventually obvious. I was to learn later that most NHS statistics cannot be relied upon.

The McNamara Fallacy is named after Robert McNamara, the US Secretary of Defence in the 1960's, who was obsessed with quantifying the Vietnam War in a way that has many parallels with NHS management today. The Vietnam War was not the US administration's finest hour!

It can be summarised as follows:-

- Measure whatever can be easily measured.

- Disregard that which cannot be measured easily.

- Presume that which cannot be measured easily is not important.

- Presume that which cannot be measured easily does not exist.

Such formalisation of assessment systems devalues the importance of judgement and intuition. The intangible cannot easily be converted into the tangible. Solving complex intangible NHS problems requires a variety of tools including clinical skills, discretionary judgement and interpersonal skills.

Kent Lodge was a purpose built, detached, specialist rehabilitation centre for the elderly built on the Broadgreen site to facilitate the closure of other isolated rehabilitation units and consolidate services. It was so-named in anticipation of being officially opened by the Duchess of Kent; unfortunately, a last minute change in schedule meant that it was in fact opened by the Duchess of Gloucester. However, the name remained. The name "Kent Lodge" was unfortunately also the home and practice address of the notorious Dr Bodkin Adams.

John Bodkin Adams (1899–1983) was a mostly private general practitioner based at Kent Lodge in Eastbourne, who was a convicted fraudster and suspected serial killer. Between 1946 and 1956, more than 160 of his patients died in circumstances which the police later thought suspicious. 132 of these patients left him money or items in their wills. {This was probably a tax avoidance scam. Instead of billing his private patients (and paying the tax on the money received) Bodkin Adams appears to have asked for legacies}. He was tried and acquitted for the murder of one patient in 1957. The trial was described at the time as "unique" because, in the words of the judge, "the act of murder" had "to be proved by expert evidence."

The trial established the doctrine of double effect, whereby a doctor giving treatment with the aim of relieving pain may, as an unintentional result, shorten life. Secondly, because of the publicity surrounding Adams's committal hearing, the law was changed to allow defendants to ask for such hearings to be held in private. Finally, though a defendant has never been required to give evidence in his own defence, the judge underlined in his summing-up that no prejudice should be attached by the jury to Adams not doing so.

Adams was found guilty in a subsequent trial of 13 offences of prescription fraud, lying on cremation forms, obstructing a police search and failing to keep a dangerous drug register. Cremation forms have a section which requires doctors to declare any pecuniary interest in the death of the deceased. He declared no such pecuniary interest. He was removed from the Medical Register in 1957 but reinstated in 1961 after two previous failed applications.

Whilst I was Clinical Director, the financial situation deteriorated. The Trust Board decided to implement a scheme to put all workers over the age of 45 on early retirement. This scheme was to be known as RAPE (retire aged person early).

Persons selected to be RAPED can apply to management to be eligible for the SHAFT scheme (special help after retirement). Persons who have been RAPED and SHAFTED will be reviewed under the SCREW scheme (scheme for retired early workers). A person may be RAPED only once, SHAFTED twice and SCREWED as many times as management deems appropriate. Persons who have been RAPED can apply to get AIDS (additional income for dependents or spouse), or HERPES (half earnings for retired personnel early severance). Obviously, persons who have AIDS or HERPES will not be SHAFTED or SCREWED any further by management. Persons staying on will receive as much SHIT (special high intensity training) as possible. Management has always prided itself about the amount of SHIT it gives its staff. Should you feel that you do not receive enough SHIT, please bring it to the attention of your manager; he has been trained to give you all the SHIT you can handle.

Life at work is like a tree full of monkeys, all on different limbs at different levels. Some monkeys are climbing up, some climbing down. The monkeys on top look down and see a tree full of smiling faces. The monkeys on the bottom look up and see nothing but assholes. When shit happens, there is usually some asshole behind it. The closer to the asshole you are the hotter the shit gets.

When stressed, it helps to remember the following prayer:

"Grant me the serenity to accept that which I cannot change, the courage to change things I cannot accept and the wisdom to hide the bodies of those people I had to kill today, because they pissed me right off".

And also "Help me to be careful of the toes I step on today, as they may be connected to the arse that I may have to kiss tomorrow".

"Help me always to give 100% at work... 12% on Monday, 23% on Tuesday, 40% on Wednesday, 20% on Thursday and 5% on Friday".

"Help me to remember that when I am having a really bad day and it seems that people are trying to piss me off, that it takes forty muscles to frown and only four to extend my arm and smack the bastard in the mouth".

The following is a list of things people would love to say out loud at work but daren't:

- I can see your point, but I still think you are full of shit.

- I don't know what your problem is, but I'll bet it's hard to pronounce.

- How about never? Is never good enough for you?

- I see you've set aside this special time to humiliate yourself in public.

- I'm really easy to get along with, once you people learn to see it my way.

- Who lit the fuse on your tampon?

- I'm out of my mind, but feel free to leave a message.

- I don't work here. I'm a consultant.

- It sounds like English but I can't understand a word you are saying.

- Ahh, I see the screwed up fairy has visited us again.

- I like you. You remind me of myself when I was young and stupid.

- You are validating my inherent mistrust of strangers.

- I have plenty of talent and vision. I just don't give a shit.

- I am already visualising the duct tape over your mouth.

- I will always cherish the initial misconception I had about you.

- Thank you. We are all refreshed and challenged by your unique point of view.

- The fact that no one understands you, doesn't mean you are an artist.

- Any resemblance between your reality and mine are purely coincidental.

- What am I? Fly paper for freaks.

- I am not being rude. You are just insignificant.

- It's a thankless job, but I have got a lot of karma to burn off.

- Yes, I am an agent of Satan but my duties are largely ceremonial.

- And your cry-baby whiney arsed opinion would be?

- Do I look like a frigging people person to you?

- This isn't an office. It's hell with fluorescent lighting.

- I started out with nothing, and I still have most of it left.

- Sarcasm is just one more service, which we offer.

- If I throw a stick, will you leave?

- Errors have been made. Others will be blamed.

- Whatever kind of look you are aiming for, you missed it.

- Oh, I get it. Like humour but different.

- An office is just a mental institute without the added walls.

- Can I swap this job for what's behind door...?

- Too many freaks, not enough circuses.

- Nice perfume (or aftershave). Must you marinate in it.

- Chaos, panic and disorder, my work here is done.

- How do I set a laser printer to stun?

- I thought I wanted a career, it turns out I just needed the money.

- I will try being nicer if you try being more intelligent.

- Wait a minute; I am trying to imagine you with a personality.

- Aren't you a black hole of need!

- I'd like to help you out, which way did you come in.

- Did you eat an extra bowl of stupidness this morning?

- Why don't you slip into something more comfortable? Like a coma.

- If you have something to say, raise your hand... then place it over your mouth.

- I'm too busy, can I ignore you some other time.

- Don't let your mind wander, it's too small to be let out on its own.

- Have a nice day, somewhere else.

- You are not yourself today, I noticed the improvement straight away.

- You are as pretty as a picture, I would really like to hang you.

- Don't believe everything you think.

- Do you hear that, that's the sound of no one caring.

Ode to the Boss.

When the body was first made, all parts wanted to be the boss.

The brain said "Since I control everything and do all the thinking, I should be the boss"

The feet said "Since I carry man where he wants to go and get in position to do what the brain wants, I should be boss"

The hands said "Since I must do all the work and earn all the money, to keep the rest of you going, I should be boss"

The eyes said "Since I must look out for all of you and tell you where danger lurks, I should be boss"

And so it went on, with the heart, the ears, the lungs etc. Finally, the arsehole spoke up and demanded that he be made the boss. All the other parts laughed at the idea of an arsehole being boss. The arsehole was so angry that he blocked himself off and refused to function. Soon, the brain was feverish, the eyes crossed and the aching feet were too weak to walk, the hand hung limply at the side and the heart and lungs struggled to function. All pleaded with the brain to relent and let the arsehole be boss! And so it happened, all the other parts did all the work and the arsehole just bossed and passed out a lot of hot shit. The moral of this story is that you do not have to be a brain to be boss, just an arsehole.

Woman

To add to the list of workplace hazardous materials, I wish to inform you of the following element, entitled 'Woman'. Its symbol is W02 and its discoverer was Adam. Its atomic mass is accepted at 118lb but is known to vary from 100lb, to 550lb. It occurs in copious quantities, in all urban areas. It has the following properties:

Physical Properties:

- Surface usually covered with a painted film.

- Boils at nothing, freezes without reason.

- Melts if given special treatment.

- Bitter if incorrectly used.

- Found in various stages, ranging from virgin metal, to common ore.

- Yields to pressure applied at correct points.

- **Chemical Properties**:

- Has great affinity for gold, silver, platinum and precious stones.

- Absorbs great quantities of expensive substances.

- May explode spontaneously, without prior warning and for no reason.

- Insoluble in liquids but activity greatly increased by saturation in alcohol.

- The most powerful money reducing agent known to man.

Common Uses:

- Highly ornamental, especially in sports cars.

- Can be a great aid to relaxation.

Tests:

- Pure specimens turn rosy pink when discovered in natural state.

- Turns green when placed near a better specimen.

Hazards:

- Highly dangerous, except in experienced hands.

- Illegal to possess more than one.

The following is a list of alternative medical terms:

Artery – the study of paintings

Bacteria – backdoor to a café

Barium – what you do with doctor's failings

Caesarean section – a district of Rome

CAT scan – searching for Kitty

Cauterise – made eye contact with her

Colic – type of sheep dog

Coma – punctuation mark

Congenital – friendly

D&C – where Washington is

Dilate – to live longer

Enema – not a friend

Genital – not Jewish

Hangnail – coat hook

High colonic – Jewish religious holiday

Impotent – distinguished and well known

Labour pain – getting hurt at work

Medical staff – doctor's walking stick

Morbid – a higher offer

Nitrate – cheaper than day rate

Node – well aware of

Outpatient – person who has fainted

PAP smear – fatherhood test

Pelvis – cousin of Elvis

Physiotherapist – exercise terrorist

Post-operative – letter carrier

Prostate – lying flat on the floor

Recovery room – place to do upholstery

Rectum – damn near killed 'em

Secretion – hiding something

Seizure – a Roman emperor

Tablet – a small table

Terminal illness – getting sick at the airport

Tibia – a country in Africa

Tumour – more than one more

Urine – opposite to your out

Varicose – nearby

Vein – conceited

When the new Clinical Director moved into his office, he found that his predecessor had provided him with two sealed envelopes. Attached to them was a note, inviting him to keep them safe but open them only if he had a serious problem.

Come the annual winter crisis, with demand exceeding supply of beds, heightened staff sickness and escalating death rate, he remembered the letters, which were conveniently labelled 1 and 2. Inside envelope 1, he found a note, saying "Blame everything on me". This traditional and well-tried management technique was effective in steering him through until the following winter crisis. Problems were even greater and death rates rose higher. He opened the second envelope. The note inside read, 'prepare two letters'.

Conundrums (with answers at the end of the book)

- The ... surgeon was ... too operate, because he had ...

The above phrase will make sense if the three blank spaces are filled by seven letters in the same order. The first space requires one word, the second space a three/four letter word and the final space a two and five letter word.

- One bright fine summer's evening, a man and his son were driving through the countryside. Upon rounding a bend, they had a head-on collision with a stationary tractor and the man was killed outright. The son was badly injured and rushed to hospital by the paramedics. On arrival in the A&E department, he was assessed by the casualty officer, whose immediate response was "My god, that's my son". The question is what was the relationship between the casualty officer and the boy?

Observations

- What did the man who first milked a cow, really think he was doing?

- Success is but failure in reverse.

- Someone must bury the undertaker.

- The only good thing about being kicked up the backside is that you must be in front.

- A prudent man is like a pin, the head prevents him going too far.

- Unlike a pregnant woman, a lightbulb can be unscrewed.

Clinical directorships are the syphilis of the NHS. They are usually acquired in unguarded moments, often leading to delusions of grandeur.

I have a theory that the fewer meetings you have, the better you do. My response to an invitation to attend meetings I considered unnecessary was to send the following by fax, and later by email:

Meetings: "Are you lonely? Work on your own? Hate making decisions? Hold a meeting! You can see other people, draw flow charts, feel important and impress your colleagues, ALL IN WORK TIME!

Meetings – the practical alternative to work.

For many managers and organisations, meetings are an end in themselves. The reason most people go to a meeting is because it is being held. A committee is mostly a gathering of important people, who singly can do nothing, but together can decide that nothing can be done. An interesting diversion in meetings is to estimate the hourly pay rate of individuals present and calculate the cost to the organisation, of holding that meeting. It normally far exceeds any potential for good.

The best meetings are one-to-one and up to three-four can be worthwhile. Once numbers exceed ten, the meetings adopt a time-wasting ritual. Any meeting lasting more than two hours is a complete waste of time. Not only has everyone's attention span waned, but if people can't decide what to do in two hours, then they all deserve the sack. Meetings are the default position for making decisions when, alternatively, a phone call or a letter would resolve the issue cheaper and often quicker.

Committee meetings reek of bureaucracy and buck passing and are rarely productive. They almost never come up with original ideas and rarely produce anything creative. It is better to do that alone and get the committee to rubber-stamp it.

The character of a chairman and the agenda content can determine how worthwhile a meeting can be. A bored chairman, with no grip on the situation, can allow the gathering to squander time on trivia and lets time be wasted on irrelevancies. A good chairman will deal with the most important matters first, whilst people are fresh and listening properly. Of course, he who writes the agenda can manipulate the proceedings to suit their personal objectives. I am told that one large firm has a meeting room with no chairs. With everyone standing up, they keep the chat to a minimum and optimise the speed of decision making.

In response to escalating average length of stay, the committee of one NHS Trust came up with an innovative solution. Basically, once they were deemed medically fit for discharge, they were served with an eviction notice and at the earliest opportunity, unceremoniously sent to a vacant nursing home bed, at their own expense. This plan was quietly shelved, after it was brought to the attention of the local press and MP.

One patient was heard to give advice to another. 'Don't mix up your Senna with your Viagra, because it will make you crap in bed'.

If you are working too hard, take 6 Senna tablets with 3 pints of beer – there is a good chance of waking up and finding yourself in a soft job.

It has been observed that it is not possible to be a little bit corrupt; it is like being a little bit pregnant. There is a village called Dull in Scotland, which has an activity centre entitled the Dull Activity Centre. The small community of Idle, near Bradford, has 'The Idle Working Man's Club'. I once saw a sign, saying 'Ears pierced while you wait'. I didn't think there was a viable alternative. Close by the hospital incinerator was a sign 'Refuse to be incinerated'. I thought I would decline too.

Many years ago, those travelling west towards Swansea on the Jersey Marine road would notice that someone had painted, on a cliff the words "Jesus Saves" under which some wag had added "Green Shield Stamps" {if you're under 50 ask a senior!}

Allegedly, Penrith train station once proudly displayed a sign on the platform urging passengers to stand well back when high speed trains passed through so as to avoid being "sucked off."

Eastbourne has more than its fair share of nursing homes catering for an ageing population. On the A22 where the road signs indicate "Newhaven for the continent" someone had unkindly added "and Eastbourne for the incontinent."

CHAPTER THIRTEEN

Medico-Legal Work

Some talented people do well because they are truly talented whilst others are simply lucky, but no-one will succeed if they fail to take opportunities when they arise. Opportunity, in the medico-legal field, knocked on my door early in my consultant career. A local solicitor, a fellow TA officer, was pursuing a case of negligence on behalf of his client – a man of 80 years who had tripped over a very uneven pavement and fractured his wrist. The orthopaedic report identified the fall as causative of the simple fracture which only needed treating with a plaster cast. The Council had a clear duty of care to maintain the pavement. They could not deny breach of that duty and consequent liability for the uneven area of pavement which they had neglected to repair despite it having been drawn to their attention months before. The man was entitled to compensation and this was not disputed. It was the amount (quantum) which was at issue. The Council noted that there was no loss of earnings involved and offered £X based upon 8-10 weeks of decreasing pain, suffering and loss of amenity (function). It was assumed that full healing of the fracture would have occurred by then with no adverse long term sequelae. I was asked to prepare a condition/prognosis report from my perspective as a geriatrician. I identified that, as is typical with the elderly, this man had been disproportionately affected. He had developed a fear of future falls and consequently had become reluctant to go out which had progressed to him becoming housebound. The knock-on effects were social isolation and depression. I estimated that in addition, his care needs had been advanced by 2 years. On the balance of probability, I gave the opinion that absent the fracture his care needs would not have reached their current level naturally due to the vicissitudes of ageing for 2 years. The judge preferred my evidence over that of the Council's expert and awarded compensation of ten times the amount originally offered. Further cases followed and slowly but surely referrals increased from further afield as I became an established expert. Criminal work, initially mostly for the police, followed as my reputation grew

Experts in general are sometimes considered to be arrogant know-alls, derided as "seagulls" swooping in from on high, crapping on those below then flying off. Some believe the word derives from ex as in "has been" and spurt as in "drip under pressure". A spoof advert probably originating in California once read "Support a lawyer, become a doctor" implying presumably that money was to be made from claims for medical negligence. In reality expert evidence from experts in a wide range of fields from accountancy through to zoology is often essential to lawyers and courts if they are to fully understand professional issues outside their own areas of expertise.

Ideally Expert Medical Witnesses should be Consultants of at least 8-10 years standing who are in active current practice. In certain specialties, especially those of a technical nature such as surgery and cardiology where things change quickly, experts can rapidly become outdated after retirement. Geriatric medicine is not so technical and after NHS retirement in 2011 I opted to continue this aspect of my practice until receipt of new instructions naturally "petered off" as time elapsed. I had expected that my currency as an expert would devalue with time. After four years this had not happened and contrary to all expectation, my work load was increasing to levels involving some 150 + new instructions per year of a mostly complex nature. Although I knew from judicial feedback, formal appraisal/feedback from SOCA (Serious Organised Crime Agency who broker police expert work nationally) and repeated instruction from major firms of solicitors (both claimant and defence), joint instruction and requests from the GMC to screen complaints that I was still well respected in my field, I elected to decline new instructions from July 2015 whilst in my prime, rather than go on and on and risk going "off the boil". (Ones reputation in the medico-legal field is constantly being informally and formally appraised with every new report by the relatively small world of experts, lawyers, coroners and judges – they do pass comment to each other without you knowing!)

Geriatric Medicine is a boom area in the medico-legal field and there is a shortage of credible experts. The primary reasons are:-

• The fear of the unknown, especially appearing in Court, discouraging new experts.

- The difficulties in balancing the needs of the case with the restrictions imposed during the day by the 2003 contract (I never signed up to this).

- Current experts are now often retired from NHS practice and are winding down.

- Referrals require a track record of medico-legal experience – no experience no referral.

There are some basic requirements over and above being expert in your field. Experts need to be able to write a report to very high standard and give an unbiased opinion to assist the courts. They need to be highly articulate in giving oral evidence and be able to think quickly on their feet when cross-examined. It helps considerably if they can impress the court by looking the part in dress and demeanour and speaking confidently. They also need to be highly organised in being able to meet deadlines and to juggle various court attendances, often across the UK. With sometimes a very early start, many Courts can be reached using the train by 10am. At any point in time experts can be asked to give their non-availability for up to 12 months! – and hold dates vacant until either a case settles or a court date is firmed up. They are essentially servants of the court and, whilst every courtesy will be potentially offered to a busy consultant the bottom line is that they can be ordered to appear as and when. Turning up late or not at all is totally unacceptable and at best will result in a judicial admonishment and/or GMC referral. In extreme cases, they may have to bear the costs of a disrupted trial or be sentenced for contempt of court. Therefore, taking on this work is not for the faint hearted or disorganised. It is however highly lucrative. The main downside is that payments are rarely prompt and sometimes solicitors insist on paying out at the end of case – which can be 2 years later. Meanwhile experts may have had to pay the tax on what was billed before receipt of any cash! It used to help to run the business as a company until the summer budget of 2015 removed the advantages.

Broadly speaking case referrals are either of a civilian nature requested by either claimant or defendant solicitors, or of a criminal nature either from the police or defendant solicitors. Independent reviews for the GMC, Trusts trying to resolve complaints without recourse to lawyers and case screenings are sometimes also requested. Reports need to be structured around liability/breach of duty, causation and current condition/ prognosis. My regular repertoire of core medical issues included bruising; CDT; delirium; dementia; dehydration; falls/fractures; pressure sores; testamentary capacity and life expectancy. I found it useful to have standard generic discussions for these key areas which I could incorporate into reports to assist the courts in understanding how I had arrived at my specific case-by-case opinions. Some negligence issues result from bad luck, minor mistakes/errors of judgement but in other cases the sheer degree of stupidity and ignorance can be truly shocking. Wilful idiocy of a reckless nature can result in criminal charges of gross negligence/manslaughter. Because of the very complex and specialised issues involved, the decision to charge doctors with criminal negligence can only be made by two highly specialised CPS units (based in York and London). They are both very slick and scrupulously fair units who were always a pleasure to advise.

The epidemic of mesothelioma, due to historic occupational asbestos contact before effective legislation reduced exposure, is just now reaching a peak as the time lag between exposure and disease can be 40 years. The main issue of causation is normally dealt with by chest physicians. However, geriatricians are becoming increasingly involved preparing reports on the peripheral issues which can represent most of the compensation "absent the mesothelioma how long would Mr X have lived and how long he would have remained fit enough to have provided care for his disabled/demented wife/widow and avoided her current care costs. Take into account and opine on Mrs X's likely trajectory of decline and her life expectancy and indicate when her needs would have exceeded his caring abilities" This is four-dimensional chess! These complex claims are normally for the order of over £500,000. Because of the high value, they are dealt with in the High Court and very able lawyers on both sides are usually involved. Opinions in these areas and on these cases, need to be handled along logical lines.

Life expectancy – The estimation of the future life expectancy of an individual is a very inexact science, regardless of the methodology employed. Actuarial tables, by the law of large numbers, allow an average life expectancy to be projected. This is the starting point. The methodology used widely by the insurance industry to determine individual risk is set out in "Medical Selection of life Risk" by R D C Brackenridge, R S Croxson and Ross McKenzie (5th Edition, 2006). However, the life expectancy of an individual is determined by a complex mix of genetic and environmental factors and chance. Perusal of records will reveal lifestyle factors, diseases or risk factors which will indicate whether life expectancy is likely to be greater or less than the average for the relevant age group cohort. Because of the high prevalence of smoking in the past, many of the risks for smoking in the elderly are already factored into the tables and may not warrant significant further discount.

Fitness – As a general rule of thumb, most elderly persons can expect that only the last third of their projected future life-expectancy will be accompanied by significant disability, with only the last few months associated with profound ill health. Light caring activities of a supervisory nature and ordinary spousal duties can usually be performed up until those last few months of profound ill health. It is only the ability to perform the heavier domestic chores and the heavier caring spousal duties (involving lifting or which are regularly accompanied by disturbed sleep) that declines in a linear manner during the last third of an elderly person's projected future life-expectancy.

Criminal cases have to be proven to the high standard of "Beyond reasonable doubt" which is 99% certainty. Most of the hassle involves the criminal work and it often pays relatively poorly at legal aid rates. The trials can drag on and experts can be kept hanging around for days at the whim of the court – Whilst the cases can be very interesting they are best declined at the outset by busy NHS Consultants. Parole board assessments sometimes provide the opportunity to visit prisons to assess a prisoner's fitness and likely risk to the public if released. Beware of these cases. One very elderly diabetic prisoner who had spent much of his adult life in prison for sex offences was considered to be at low risk of repetition and released on licence. He obtained a private prescription for Viagra from a GP unaware of his background and resumed his offending. He spent the rest of his days behind bars. Prison categories are:

- CATEGORY A – For prisoners deemed to be of risk to the public and/or with the desire and support/means (possibly external) to escape.

- CATEGORY B – For prisoners at high escape risk but lacking the means and support to so do.

- CATEGORY C – For prisoners not at high escape risk but who could be opportunists.

- CATEGORY D – For prisoners of no risk to the public and of no escape risk.

Visiting a prisoner needs to be planned well in advance and permission of the Governor obtained – get the solicitor to do this. All prisons have very tight security checks on visitors – including doctors. Try to carry as little as possible – stethoscope, pen and paper is all you need – other bits of medical equipment will be available in the prison medical centre. Anything deemed contraband or unnecessary will not be allowed in. Do you leave stuff (mobile, money, house keys, handbag) in the car? I always consider car parks for prison visitors (which are never actually close to the prison gates) to be the potentially most dangerous places to park. They tend to be frequented by the criminal fraternity who can be opportunists! Female doctors are advised to look and dress as plainly as possible.

Civilian cases have to be proven to the lesser standard of "balance of probability" which is more than 51% certainty. These cases rarely actually get to court as most are settled by agreement/compromise to avoid the loser bearing the costs of the trial. The conduct of these cases is governed by very strict part 35 rules which apply both to lawyers and experts. They dictate tight time-frames for all and cases can be thrown out if one side is deemed to be "timed-out". Experts must give unbiased evidence for the Court and not evidence biased to one side. Almost all these civilian cases stand or fall on the quality of the expert evidence. Clever and creative lawyering moves can seriously wrong-foot experts. The classic trick is for the claimant's solicitor to disclose all the evidence (as they must) but in a large bundle (2-3000 sheets) of disorganised and often irrelevant records in the hope that the single page of evidence damaging to a claimant's case will be missed by the defendant's expert. It is not unheard of for them to photocopy everything else twice, shuffle it and randomly insert that one page. If the expert misses it, it's the expert's fault. Experts need to know what ought to be there and look for it. If it's not there then comment upon the absence! There are, however, lots of other clever legal moves along the way which can hassle experts by leaving the deadlines short.

- The need for a meeting (on the phone normally) with the other side's expert to set out areas of agreement and disagreement in a joint report − normally the claimant's expert is the scribe.

- Answering questions posed by both sides.

- Having to hold dates vacant in case of a trial. Each side will try to gain the upper hand through their expert being more available than the opposition.

Coroner work normally comes on the back of an initial report for the police which have found insufficient grounds for criminal charges. Sometimes Coroners commission their own reports when the case is controversial. Coroners run their own fiefdoms and standards vary. Technically an Inquest is held to establish the cause of death by answering the questions − who, what, how, when and where (but not the why) if the death may not, at first sight, be due to natural causes. An inquest conclusion is based upon "balance of probability" and ought not to apportion blame in a way which could be used by other courts in a negligence claim. Some coroners will determine cause of death without recourse to an inquest. Others will give a family with grievances their time in court. This inevitably results in the interested parties being "lawyered up" including typically –the family, the Hospital Trust, the GP and the Community Trust if there has been DN input. Thus 4 solicitors each accompanied by a barrister will be present and eager to ask questions. These inquests can drag on as the issues expand if the Coroner fails to get a grip. Inquests involving industrial accidents, health and safety issues and deaths in custody must have a jury but the Coroner can summon a jury in any cases.

Most doctors at some point in their career will be subject to a GMC complaint. These are often malicious, unfounded complaints which lead nowhere. They are screened out by expert opinion early in the process. The bottom line is that they go nowhere if the doctor's standard has merely fallen below, but not seriously below, standard as a one-off. Any attempt at the cover-up of an honest mistake or error of judgment almost always results in standards being deemed to be "seriously below standard". In that event trouble looms.

Appearing in court is an alien concept to most people and the run up to a trial can generate considerable anxiety. Doctors can appear in any of the three categories of witness. Witness to fact – they just happen to be doctors who have witnessed something happening which is unrelated to their job. Professional witness – describing what they saw and did in their professional role, often treating the injuries following an accident or assault. Expert witnesses normally have had no active professional role but are asked to give an opinion after the event – they are the only witnesses who can give opinion under oath, everyone else is limited to outlining what they saw and did. Facts are for courts, not experts, to determine. It is not uncommon for experts to have to give alternative opinions depending upon which facts the courts determine to be true.

A typical criminal case, involving a medical expert, will have been investigated by the police and that evidence reviewed by the expert whose opinion will be crucial when submitted to the CPS for a decision as to whether to prosecute. The expert's contact details will be passed to "Witness Care" who will update them on the pre-trial progress and give due warning of the trial date. They will be your principle contact, though the CPS Solicitors may have met with you to check out your degree of certainty about your opinion – they will want no surprises in court. The CPS will then appoint a barrister to prosecute. The role of the prosecution is to build an unassailable wall of evidence. The role of the defence is to breach it thereby causing the jury to have reasonable doubt. They may have their own expert whose opinion is likely to contradict yours. Experts ought to have seen each other's reports and commented thereon before the trial. Perfect planning prevents pathetic performance. On the day of the trial there are some "tips" which, if followed, prevent problems:-

- Double check your report for any stupid errors or inconsistencies and re-evaluate whether you are still of the same opinion. Take a copy with you.

- Decide early what you will be wearing. A suit is expected but it ought to be comfortable, tidy and preferably not brand new. It ought to be the sort of suit that the judge and barristers wear, not the sort that a defendant might have bought from the supermarket two days earlier.

- Decide how you will be travelling (avoid driving on the day-hold-ups will wrong foot you badly) and whether on the same day or the night before and organise train tickets early to avoid queuing. Early morning trains are generally very reliable. There is a fairly high chance that on these early trains, one of your fellow passengers will be a barrister, judge or witness who could be involved in your trial – so keep your own counsel. If travelling the day before, witness care will sort out accommodation but remember that other guests may also have involvement in your trial.

- Make sure that you have had a good breakfast – lunch breaks are rarely before 1pm and not all courts have canteens.

- Always arrive at court earlier than you were told. There is "airport security" to pass through. Then report to an usher. If you are a "Crown witness", witness care will be alerted and look after you. There will be normally be a room exclusively for prosecution witnesses with tea, coffee, water and toilets – use the former sparingly and the latter frequently. You ought to be kept informed as to progress and when you are likely to be called. As a Crown witness you cannot discuss the case with other witnesses or hear any evidence until after yours is given. If you are a defence witness the usher might alert the defence team to your arrival but you will basically be left to your own devices and have to sit in the public areas with the criminal fraternity who will not be hard to identify. (The really scruffy ones carrying a hold-all and wearing a face like a robber's dog are expecting to be sent directly to gaol upon sentencing). You are best checking the court, listing and lurking near the allocated courtroom in the hope that you can catch the eye of one of the defence team. Defence witnesses can sit in court throughout and will usually be sat behind defence counsel and expected to advise them on awkward questions to pose of prosecution experts.

- Check whether the judge is "your honour" or "your lordship" in case you need to address them directly. The longer the wig, the more red and frills in the robes are good indicators of seniority.

- Make the usher aware as to whether you wish to swear an oath or affirm. When your time comes use this to test the acoustics of the courtroom.

- Give your evidence standing not sitting. Not only does this look more professional but it keeps you more alert. Position yourself comfortably so as to face the judge and jury – they are the only important ones. Turn head and shoulders to receive questions from barristers but turn back to the comfy position to deliver answers facing the judge and jury.

- If you are a "Crown witness" you will be called early in the trial to give your evidence "in chief" to assist prosecuting counsel in building their wall of evidence. You will be controlled very tightly as you are taken carefully through your report – yes or no answers will probably be all that they want.

Stick to that unless told otherwise. Giving evidence 'in chief' could well take an hour or so.

- Immediately afterwards, and normally without a break, you will be subject to cross-examination by the defence counsel. This could be another couple of hours. They will aim to discredit your evidence and opinion.

- Beware of the over pleasant approach. That normally means that they are confident about leading you to a position which suits their client. If the questions become aggressive you are probably doing a better job than was expected.

- Be on your guard for some classic ploys.

- The prefatory statement will be phrased "I am sure that you are aware of the important work of Prof. Jones in this area. Could you then please tell me why your opinion...." Now you are potentially in trouble! You have either heard of Prof. Jones and his work or not. If you have never heard of him and he is truly important your credibility in the eyes of the jury will falter if you admit your ignorance. There will be strong temptation to "blank" the bit about Prof. Jones. If you do you have effectively agreed that he is important – leaving the way open for his ideas, however eccentric, to be introduced and undermine your evidence. It is better to admit ignorance of his work on the basis that if he was that important in your field of expertise you would have heard of him and his work. If you are right counsel will move on. If you are wrong and he is the world authority you're stuffed especially if he is the one sitting in court advising the defence team.

- A good defence counsel can slowly by degrees move you into a position where they can suddenly demand an inappropriately simple yes or no answer to a very complex issue. If you failed to see it coming all you can do is appeal to the judge for a ruling on the basis that there is a danger that you could mislead the court by giving too simple an answer to complex issues.

- After cross-examination and hopefully after a break for lunch, prosecution counsel will again have their turn to quiz you to reverse any perceived damage to their case.

- Normally after giving your evidence you will have the opportunity to hear the expert evidence put forward by the defence.

Civilian cases of negligence normally start with proving liability to provide a duty of care. For bodies such as the NHS, Nursing Homes, and Councils the duty of care cannot normally be denied. The next step is proving that there was a breach of that duty of care according to the "Bolam Standard" – Where clinical negligence is claimed, the Bolam test is the one used to determine the standard of care owed by professionals to those whom they serve, e.g. the standards of care provided to patients by doctors. The case Bolam v Friern Hospital Management Committee (1957) established that if a doctor acts in accordance with a responsible body of medical opinion, he or she will not be negligent. The Bolam Principle is clear that the standard of care must be judged by the standards of a practitioner of the same specialty and the same grade. This is because practitioners from differing specialties will have different knowledge and experience and this leads to differences in approach, in potential awareness of risk, and a different differential diagnosis for any clinical situation.

Many have heard of the Bolam test without knowing the full background. The full details, as described in Wikipedia were:-

{Mr Bolam was a voluntary patient at a mental health institution run by the Friern Hospital Management Committee. He agreed to undergo electro-convulsive therapy. He was not given any muscle relaxant, and his body was not restrained during the procedure. He flailed about violently before the procedure was stopped, and he suffered some serious injuries, including fractures of the acetabula (hip). He sued the Committee for compensation. He argued they were negligent for

- Not issuing relaxants.

- Not restraining him.

- Not warning him about the risks involved.

McNair J at the first instance noted that expert witnesses had confirmed, that much medical opinion was opposed to the use of relaxant drugs, and that manual restraints could sometimes increase the risk of fracture. Moreover, it was the common practice of the profession to not warn patients of the risk of treatment (when it is small) unless they are asked. He held that what was common practice in a particular profession was highly relevant to the standard of care required. A person falls below the appropriate standard, and is negligent, if he fails to do what a reasonable person would in the circumstances. But when a person professes to have professional skills, as doctors do, the standard of care must be higher. "It is just a question of expression," said McNair J.

In this case, the verdict was in favour of the defendant hospital. Given the general medical opinions about what was acceptable electro-shock practice, they had not been negligent in the way they carried out the treatment}

Subsequently, this standard of care test was amended – the Bolitho amendment – to include the requirement that the doctor should also have behaved in a way that 'withstands logical analyses regardless of the body of medical opinion'. The determination of whether a professional's actions or omissions withstand logical analysis is the responsibility of the court.

Having established duty of care and breach of duty, the next step is to identify the consequences – what that breach of duty caused. The final step is quantifying the adverse consequences. General pain, suffering and loss of amenity will be worthy of compensation by way of general damages. These may be as special damages worthy of a claim for specific areas of detriment.

It is estimated that every year more than 1 million patients and care home residents suffer avoidable harm. Some 5.6% of patients suffered from serious and avoidable bedsores. Falls are the next most frequent cause of avoidable harm. The classic trip hazards at home are cats, mats and dressing gowns. The latter are often old, warm, well-loved and long-reaching to just above the ankle. Gradual loss of height from osteoporosis results in dressing gowns reaching the floor and causing falls.

In hospitals and care homes the frail but mobile elderly mostly fall near beds or in bathrooms whilst transferring position and the actual fall is rarely witnessed. Falls from beds are common. Serious injuries can result which can be lethal or life-changing.

Fracture to the hip in the older person is a devastating life event, associated with significant mortality and morbidity. Up to a third of those sustaining such fractures die within 12 months. Of those who survive with normal cognitive function, only 50% gain independence but often to a level of function below that which they enjoyed before the fracture. In the presence of dementia, the majority of the survivors are left with such a degree of disability, that independent living is impossible, and they enter residential or nursing homes.

Even minor head injuries can have serious consequences. Subdural haematomas are collections of blood clot in the subdural space within the skull but outside the brain. This space contains bridging veins and a slow venous bleed may result spontaneously or more usually from head injury if the veins rupture. Brain atrophy (shrinkage) which accompanies great age puts these veins under tension increasing the risk of rupture. The resistance of the vein walls to tears also deteriorates with age. As a result, subdural haematomas are common in the elderly and typically present some days or even weeks (depending on a number of factors including the rate of bleed/ooze) after a trivial and often unremembered head injury. The venous ooze may cease early and result in only a small collection which can be easily accommodated around an atrophic brain. These can be asymptomatic. More usually the clot expands slowly eventually causing neurological signs as the brain is squeezed. Some smaller clots can stabilise and resolve with time and are managed conservatively. Others require burr hole drainage to remove the clot. Aspirin and warfarin increase both the risk and rate of bleeding and deterioration can be rapid.

Brisk bleeding from anticoagulation will only cease when the clot has expanded such as to raise the pressure within the skull sufficiently above venous pressure. Inevitably the brain will be severely squeezed. Rapid deterioration in levels of consciousness and large clots are bad prognostic signs and are normally a harbinger of death. Older individuals, even if not frail, lack the physiological reserve (stamina) to recover from neurosurgery and generally fare badly. There is a very high perioperative mortality rate. If they survive the immediate aftermath of neurosurgery there is often severe residual brain damage and older patients rarely return to anything approaching previous levels of function. Full time care in a nursing home is very often required. It is thus common for Neurosurgeons to decline to operate in "the best interests of the patient" when the prognosis for meaningful recovery is very poor.

Falls – The upright human being is intrinsically unstable. Falls in the young and fit are rare, simply because good eyesight, efficient hearing and normal sensation in the limbs give early warning of environmental hazards, which are compensated for by suppleness of the limbs, muscular strength and a brain, which is quick to act, to alter bodily position accordingly. By contrast, failing eyesight, deafness and decreased sensation in the limbs make the frailer older person less aware of their surroundings and reaction to normal hazards is impeded by decrease in muscular strength, arthritis and slow brain functioning – partly the result of the normal aging process, which is made even worse in the presence of dementia. Paradoxically, the slower walking gait, which comes with ageing, enhances the tendency to fall. Even in the best institutions, falls can never be entirely prevented without so restricting patient autonomy to a degree which would constitute abuse. However, the preventative measures as recommended by NICE Guideline CG161 can reduce the likelihood of falls, especially in the absence of dementia or confusion. Those measures are less successful when there is confusion because such patients undertake risky manoeuvres and may not remember to summon assistance.

Cot sides – The use of restraints and cot sides/bed rails in institutions is controversial and opinions as to the wisdom of their use have varied over the years. There is no doubt that they prevent small accidental falls in unwell restless patients but on the other hand, confused and agitated individuals may see them as a challenge and in attempting to climb over them, risk more serious injury. The assessment of risk/benefit in the use of cot sides is very subjective and can and often does change day by day. Pressure alert mats can give warning of the imminent potential for a fall from bed but can only prevent falls if the staff are vigilant.

The other main causes of harm were urinary tract infections linked with catheter use, blood clots and poor monitoring of anticoagulants. Drug errors, including giving the correct dose to the wrong patient, whilst common, rarely cause serious problems. Figures released by the NHS Litigation Authority (NHSLA) on legal costs for the four year period ending in 2014 indicated the payment of some £502m to just ten top law firms including damages and costs. Whilst the Government is trying to reduce the legal costs, claimant legal firms claim that their costs consistently amount to less than 10% of the compensation secured for claimants. They also indicate that the costs could be kept low if the NHSLA admitted liability earlier in the process in clear cut cases instead of defending them.

EPILOGUE

This book is primarily dedicated to my dear wife Linda, whose unfailing support through the thick and thin of life, since we met in 1973, has been above and beyond the call of wifely duty. In retrospect, she has had to put up with some of my occasional, short-lived but extreme eccentricities, in addition to my normal extrovert traits. When working from home, I can be extremely focussed on the task in hand, to the point of rudeness if interrupted, and generally oblivious to the normal social courtesies expected. For some years, she thought that I was becoming deaf as I often failed to heed some of her requests. When I repeatedly failed to arrange hearing tests, she booked one for me a few months ago. To keep the peace, I attended with good grace, only to find that there was minimal loss, consistent with the vicissitudes of normal ageing. I had been exposed as "choice deaf". Some cases have resulted in major domestic upheaval – the following are worth a mention:-

- The arrival of 118Kg of documents in 8 large boxes took over the house for weeks before the key material was identified and the report written.

- Over one weekend I was in charge of the original records (two large suitcases worth) of some 50 living individuals whilst they were sorted and photocopied. Had any of them been taken ill over that period I was the primary reference point for any doctor who needed background information. The judge ordered that they could not leave my side. Fortunately, the process was accomplished quickly when the large Manchester firm of solicitors opened their office specially and brought in a team of secretaries to use four industrial sized photocopying machines. In two days, all the records were copied, paginated into a master copy and then a further 12 copies made.

- The outcome of one high value civilian case rested heavily on my evidence. Unfortunately, the case was scheduled for 10.30 am in Manchester on the Tuesday when we were due to arrive at Heathrow airport from Cape Town at 6.30 am. It was just do-able but only by using either chartered helicopter or private limo (at their client's expense). This was potentially highly disruptive – not only did I have to lug my "Court suit" on holiday in readiness and face a few hours giving evidence after a poor night's sleep, but also Linda had to anticipate a few hours of abandonment in Manchester with all our luggage until I was released. As it worked out, I was informed by fax on the Monday morning that the case had settled and my presence was unnecessary.

Linda, thank you for your forbearance.

Our three daughters, Emma, Jessica and Georgina also deserve a serious mention for their encouragement and tolerance over the years. Sons tend to cut the apron strings and when they get married, focus upon their new families. Daughters, however, tend to remain more in touch with their roots and parents. When active retirement morphs through inactivity to dependency, daughters are "the guards". They need to be kept on side. One widower's caring daughter took matters too far. She lived next door to him and installed a "plug in" baby monitor to listen out for trouble. When it went silent at 11pm, she rushed around letting herself in quietly, expecting the worst. He had in fact switched it off whilst bonking his new lady friend. Neither female was impressed!

In addition to thanking friends for their encouragements, special thanks are owed to my secretary/PA, Mrs Patricia Hunt, for her efficiencies, suggestions, speed and accuracy in typing up and finalising my medico-legal reports. Pat has done this over many years, as well as assisting in creating and typing this book.

No doctor works in isolation and over my career, I have been supported by Consultant colleagues, junior doctors and numerous members of the nursing profession, both senior and junior. Many have provided material which expanded the archive from which this book was written. Numerous sources available on the internet, particularly Wikipedia have allowed me to "flesh out" some issues. I thank you all.

This work is now effectively finished, along the lines envisaged. It has remained light-hearted, with bits of seriousness, intended to appeal to the general public. I originally planned to round it off with a succession of chapters of a more serious, technical and detailed nature, describing some more of my medico-legal cases and the appropriate law. On reflection, I decided that this would, be inappropriate to include in a book of humour.

However, that serious unused material has proved more than adequate to generate a second book provisionally entitled "The Geriatrician in Court" which is structured to provide comprehensive advice on a medico-legal career. As such it is packed with practical advice on appearing in court with numerous casework examples on how expert conclusions were reached, and why.

Enough is enough for now. To avoid embarrassment to family members, I have mostly refrained from including exposés from the domestic front but on reflection and in the spirit of the book, some brief anecdotes are worth a mention:-

- Canine roundworms can cause diseases in humans (Toxocariasis). Worm eggs are excreted in dog faeces and after two weeks in the environment, they become infectious to humans. If accidentally ingested, the worms can migrate to organs like the liver, lungs, brain and eyes. Because of the necessary two week incubation period, your child is minimally at risk if found to be eating a fresh dog turd.

- Teenage girls go through a period whereby they are attracted to males with the opposite traits to their fathers. Be prepared to meet a succession of uncouth, barely articulate youths, who lack the vestiges of social graces. One bunch of testosterone fuelled persistent visitors were nicknamed "Robin Hood and his Merry Men". Fortunately, most grow out of it quickly and end up settling down with someone similar to you.

- Delight in the noisy chatterboxes, even though your phone bill will rise. They are training for either politics, the Bar or teaching. The aim appears to be able to talk non-stop for an hour, without saying a great deal. I once overheard two young men at a party (clearly seeking refuge from Miss Chatterbox), commenting that possibly the best thing about oral sex with her, would be 10 minutes of peace and quiet. I was so amused that I couldn't resist introducing myself – much to their embarrassment!

- When asked in a coffee shop what STD stood for, I carefully outlined the dangers of unprotected sex not realising that the question was prompted by the price list for std, med and lge coffees. However, I shall absolutely refrain from relating any anecdotes from the golf club, grand parenting and active retirement for fear of sullying matters. I shall depend on these for the future. There are seriously keen and able golfers – I should not be included within their number. I enjoy long walks around the course following the ball, which has often neither achieved the distance or direction intended. I live in hope that with more time to practice, improvement will follow. I am at the watershed between giving up medicine and the unknown planet of the future. Everything has a reason and the wisdom of my decision to decline future new medico-legal instructions was reinforced by two developments, not of my making:-

- Changes were announced in the July 2015 budget, to take effect from April 2016, which will significantly reduce the advantages of running a business as a limited company. The Government believes the way dividends are taxed currently –

including the dividend tax credit – is "arcane" and "complex" and the Chancellor believes that many people now work via their own limited companies, simply to save tax, i.e. 'tax motivated incorporation'. From April 2016, notional 10% tax credit on dividends will be abolished. A £5,000 tax free dividend allowance will be introduced. Dividends above this level will be taxed at 7.5% (basic rate), 32.5% (higher rate), and 38.1% (additional rate). This is in addition to the corporation tax of 21% – I refer you to the "Laffer Curve"!

- The General Medical Council (GMC) controls and regulates the practice of Medicine in the UK. Their current slogan on all their communications reads "*Working with doctors, working for patients*". To practise medicine in the UK, doctors need to be both registered with the GMC and hold a licence to practise. (Technically a licence is unnecessary to write medico-legal reports, though some instructing lawyers require it and the medical defence organisations require one to hold a licence, if preparing condition and prognosis reports, as patients (though technically they are clients) need to be seen and examined). However, no expert would wish to have their competence to give evidence in court tarnished, by lack of a licence, so most have retained one). Retention of one's licence is dependent upon demonstrating competence within one's field of practise. This requires proof of the achievement of continuous professional development (CPD), 365 degree feedback and demonstration of competence at annual appraisal. Every 5 years the process is

272

more formal, involving revalidation of one's fitness to retain a licence, based upon those annual appraisals. For doctors in employment, this is straightforward and done by a Responsible Officer or Suitable Person – normally the medically qualified clinical director or medical director. For those in independent practice, such as myself, it was more complex. Nonetheless, I jumped through all the hoops after 2011 and was revalidated in July 2015, expecting it to be for the standard five year term. I was therefore surprised to receive this letter.

"I'm writing to tell you that from January 2016, we're introducing a revalidation assessment for certain groups of licensed doctors. This affects you because you have told us that you don't have a connection to a Responsible Officer or Suitable Person, who can make a revalidation recommendation about you. All licensed doctors who do not have a Responsible Officer or Suitable Person must sit an assessment and reach the required standard, before we can agree their revalidation.

Why must I sit an assessment?

As a licensed doctor without a connection, you need to sit this assessment to show your medical knowledge is up to date. We will consider your performance in the assessment, together with all of the other evidence you have submitted to us, as part of the annual return process, to determine whether you should retain your licence to practise and be revalidated.

The Assessment

The revalidation assessment will be a single written 'multiple choice' test of knowledge, comprising 120 single best answer questions. It's designed to test a doctor's ability to apply their knowledge to the care of patients in the UK.

You can choose from 11 available assessments, each one covering a primary medical specialty, such as General Practice or Paediatrics. There will also be one assessment available that is generic in nature, rather than specialty specific. All assessments will take place at our Clinical Assessment Centre in Manchester, UK.

The fee to sit the assessment is £1100. This charge is based on recovering the full cost of delivering the assessment from those who need to take it.

When do I need to sit my assessment?

We'll give you four months' notice to book a place to sit your assessment. You'll need to use GMC Online to do this and pay the fee when you make your booking. Assessment places are spread throughout the year. You should choose the next available convenient date for the assessment, in your chosen practice area.

From January 2016 onwards, we'll start writing to those doctors who will need to sit an assessment. You can expect to receive your booking notice before the end of 2016. Failure to sit an assessment when asked to do so may put your licence to practise at risk. In the meantime, you must continue to have regular appraisals and complete your online annual returns, when we ask you to do so. From January 2016, a fee of £250 will be payable when you submit an annual return".

Fortunately, neither the GMC changes nor the tax changes will affect me and in due course I shall voluntarily relinquish both my registration and licence. Traditionally, many doctors, even after total retirement, would remain on the register for a few years. For some, it was to hedge their bets in case of being asked to do the odd locum. For most however, it was altruistic, such that they could serve their fellow man in the event of a national crisis. In the event of past crises, retired doctors have been a useful resource – available to take on many of the vital but non-clinical backroom roles (e.g. signing death certificates etc.), thus releasing those still in practice, for the more important work of treatment. Sadly, this is positively being discouraged.

The answer to the first conundrum in chapter 12 is notable; not able and no table. The relationship between the boy and doctor was that she was his mother. When I first heard this in the mid 70's so few doctors in A&E were female that almost no-one worked it out!

I am told that the reason that demons hang around with ghouls on Halloween is that demons are a girl's best friend! I shall finish off with the following anagrams, as yet unused: supernatural – usual partner; gargoyle – royal egg; moisten – one mist; maine – I name; hour being – neighbour; platinum – lamp unit; tension – one isn't; lemonade – meal done. Finally, naughtiness (is known) as eight nuns.

Farewell!